Heart 2 Heart

*Stories from Patients with
Left Ventricular Assist Devices*

D0862886

Edited by

Ruth Halben, M.S.W.

Lake Michigan Sunset
Cover photography by G. Randall Goss
Reprinted with permission

Cover Design by Aki Yao and Marissa Rivas Taylor
Learning Design & Publishing
Health Information Technology and Services
University of Michigan

Produced by Learning Design & Publishing
Health Information Technology and Services
University of Michigan

Published by Michigan Publishing
University of Michigan Library

ISBN: 978-1-60785-398-5

Dedication

Hope. Anticipation. Fear. Excitement. Anger. A sense of purpose. Denial. Joy. Boredom. Gratitude. Love of family. Contemplating death. The will to live. Acceptance. Life comes into sharper focus in times of personal challenge. In these pages, women and men with severe heart failure whose lives have been forever altered by the experience of living first with advanced heart failure and then a ventricular assist device (VAD) share their emotional stories.

This remarkable therapy allows us to cheat death, sometimes for many years, in patients previously at the precipice. For most patients, quality of life on a VAD is remarkably good. However, complications – stroke, life-threatening infections, gastrointestinal bleeding and the need for heart pump replacement - remain all too common. Their capacity to adjust to these changing life circumstances, to accept the restored opportunities afforded by VAD therapy along with the emotional burden of knowing that any day could bring tragedy, is testament to the amazing resilience and adaptability that makes us human.

As a cardiologist working with patients with advanced heart failure, I have been privileged to bear witness to the spirit of those who have pioneered the first two decades of widely-available ventricular assist device therapy, sharing in their joys and disappointments, their challenges and their triumphs. These reflections open that experience to a much wider audience. In 2016, to receive a ventricular assist device remains an uncommon experience; the emotional lives of those who do so are universal.

Keith Aaronson, M.D., M.S.
Bertram Pitt, M.D. Collegiate Professor of Cardiovascular Medicine
Professor of Internal Medicine
Medical Director, Heart Transplant Program and Center for Circulatory Support
University of Michigan
Ann Arbor, MI

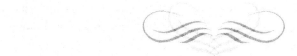

Contents

Foreword

From a very basic scientific description, heart failure is the inability of the heart to pump blood commensurate with the needs of the body. The causes of heart failure are varied, stemming from something as common as a heart attack to something less common, such as a genetic defect in the muscle of the heart.

This simplistic scientific description of heart failure ignores the staggering toll of human limitations and suffering caused by heart failure as it progresses from its earliest stages to more advanced states. In its worst form, heart failure causes painful swelling of the body, extreme fatigue, chest pains, dizziness and extreme shortness of breath with little or no activity. These symptoms prevent participation in even the simplest activities of daily living such as bathing, brushing one's teeth or dressing. For some, sleeping in an upright position in a chair helps prevent their lungs from drowning in their own fluids.

Why is it important to understand the human suffering caused from heart failure? In the upcoming pages of this book you are going to hear stories from patients and families about their experiences and decisions to accept one treatment option for heart failure.

The treatment, a left ventricular assist device or LVAD, is an artificial heart pump that is attached to the heart through a major surgical operation that takes over the pumping action of the left side of the heart to relieve the symptoms of heart failure. Over the past 30 years, LVADs have moved from being a rarity to now becoming the most common forms of treatment for severe advanced cases of heart failure for those that are eligible and choose to accept this treatment.

For the very late stages of heart failure, scientific evidence strongly suggests that LVADs provide survival benefit and an improvement in one's quality of life. Technological improvements in LVADs have reduced their size from that of a grapefruit to that of a plum. In fact, LVADs have now become more common than heart transplantation because of the scarce limitations in heart donors.

Many wonder at the marvels of man being able to create a machine that to some extent, replicates the exquisite human function of the heart. However, the story is not so simple. LVADs, despite all the marvels and benefits they possess, have an ugly side to them and are associated with a host of complications including stroke, bleeding, infection and blood clots forming in the heart pump that may occur in some patients at a not too infrequent rate.

The stories in this book describe the difficult dilemma that patients face in trying to decide to accept a life-altering therapy that relieves the unimaginable suffering of advanced stages of heart failure, but for some may cause a series of dreadful or potentially deadly complications.

After reading these stories, one should marvel not at the life-saving technology of the LVAD, but at the strength and the capacity of our patients to endure. The stories describe the human spirit at its greatest when facing both the joys that LVAD therapy can bring and its darkest hours. These stories are about patients making a choice between life and death. All of these patients are brave, both in life and as they approach death.

Francis Pagani, M.D., Ph.D.
Otto Gago, M.D. Professor of Cardiac Surgery
University of Michigan Frankel Cardiovascular Center
Surgical Director, Heart Transplant Program and Center for Circulatory Support
University of Michigan
Ann Arbor, MI

Preface

In the spring of 1996, as a graduate student at University of Michigan's School of Social Work, I was in my second semester at University Hospital in the Heart and Lung Transplant Programs. My preceptor thought it would be 'very interesting' for me to organize a group of patients and teach them leadership skills in order to better facilitate the patient run support groups that she had started throughout Michigan. Her suggestion was based on my former work experience as an Advertising Manager and Director of Sales for a large publishing company. Plus, she thought I should take a class in 'group therapy.' To be honest, I wasn't very interested in groups for reasons too numerous to list here. However, under her influence, I signed up for the class and extended an invitation to the group leaders she provided.

On our first meeting, I quickly learned that these individuals already had leadership skills; they were experts in their own illness and treatments. They immediately challenged me to help them put on a conference to include all transplant patients in Michigan. Their vision was a statewide affair with speakers from many areas of health care: insurance companies, legislators, doctors and more. After several months of planning, the conference was successfully held with over 500 patients and their families in attendance.

During one of the presentations, a pre-transplant lung patient stood up and shared that she wasn't sure her life was worth putting her family through the expense, both emotional and financial, to have a transplant. She was in tears as all those present heard her breath-shortened plea. That's when Pat, a heart recipient, stood up. Pat was a regular member of our support group and had quite a way with words. She asked all who thought this woman was 'worth it' to stand in support. The entire assembly rose to their feet and applauded, including the panel of speakers who were presenting at that moment.

I can't tell you how moved I was by this demonstration of sharing and support. It was sincere and heartfelt. In that brief question, this woman had told her story, one of suffering and fear about the future. Also in that moment, she received support from many others who'd likely felt like her at one time or another. And now through this conference, they were sharing and learning from not only the 'experts,' but from each other. For me, that conference was the inspiration for this book and the catalyst for many other programs developed in support of heart transplants, and eventually LVAD patients and their families at University of Michigan Hospital.

During my twenty-one years as a professional social worker, I have learned much about the benefits of peer-to-peer support. The group that I helped facilitate during my internship still endures as a resource for new patients, those waiting and those who have undergone LVAD or heart transplant surgeries. Our 'Peer Visitors' are mentors, trained to meet with other patients, either in the hospital or out. Each year two large social events are hosted by social work so that patients can connect or reconnect with others and share their experiences. A newsletter of patient events is published each quarter to keep the patients and their families informed of the heart transplant and LVAD happenings. And, once each year, with each patient's permission, a directory is published and given to every patient in our program so that they may 'resource' one another by phone, letter or email. These activities are self-supported by an annual hockey game fundraiser.

The power of shared experiences is well documented in literature on story telling. The stories told in this book contain personal accounts of high points, low points and turning points of emotionally charged events. They have helped make meaning out of suffering and setbacks not only for their writers, but also for those of us who read them. This book is a culmination of efforts that will hopefully help inform future patients in their decision making about having and living with an LVAD. And, more importantly, encourage them to share their experience; to tell their story to a doctor, nurse, social worker, family member and each other.

Ruth Halben, B.A., M.S.W.

Acknowledgements

It is with deepest gratitude, I'd like to thank:

My **Dad**, who always told me that I could do anything.

My **children** and **their wonderful families,** who are the very best part of me.

My daughter **Andrea**, whose time on earth was so limited but she made such a big impact.

Oliva Alban Kuester, M.S.W., for her mentorship and excellence in teaching me how to take the classroom into the field.

Erica Perry, M.S.W., for teaching me the art of group and peer support.

Joan Meagher, B.S.N., for teaching me the fundamentals of excellence in patient care.

Maureen Daly, B.S.N., for her practical contribution to this work but more for her own excellence in LVAD patient care.

Monica Johnson, B.S.N., M.S.A. whose coordination efforts are so very much appreciated.

Erin Spangler, M.S.W. my work partner in VAD social work, who has helped on this project in a variety of ways and is just an amazing co-worker and social worker.

Dawn Shufflin, Administrative Coordinator and Project Coordinator for Cardiac Surgery who sees to so many details and makes our program 'go.'

Graduate students who have been my interns as well as the undergraduate *Health Science Scholars* and those students who have volunteered in our program, you have all taught me so much.

G. Randal Goss, my very talented brother-in-law for the book cover photo but also for all of his professional photographic contributions to our family over the years

Jasna Markovac, Ph.D., Senior Director, Learning Design and Publishing, Health Information Technology and Services, University of Michigan, for her encouragement and steadfastness when this project stalled.

Marissa Rivas Taylor, M.S., Publishing Editor, Learning Design and Publishing, Health Information Technology and Services, University of Michigan, for her careful listening and help in bringing this project to its conclusion.

Keith Aaronson, M.D., Medical Director of the University of Michigan Heart Transplant Program and Center for Circulatory Support, for his unwavering understanding of the importance of social work's role in heart transplantation and LVAD implantation.

Francis D. Pagani, M.D., Ph.D. Surgical Director of Heart Transplantation and Director of the Center for Circulatory Support at University of Michigan, without whom there would be no LVAD program and consequently I would not have returned to the University of Michigan, nor would I have seen an actual heart transplant. You are, of course, a very accomplished surgeon. But many may not know that you were the inspiration for a 15-year-old hockey fundraiser, for which many other professionals have learned the joy of skating in order to support it as well. Thank you for the opportunity of a lifetime to work with you as you built this world class LVAD program. Thank you for your contribution to this book; for your much needed travel support over these many years; and finally for your recognition and support of the role of social work and understanding the importance of social support in all of its many facets.

And lastly but never least, the **patients** and **their caregivers**, not just those who have bravely shared their stories here but those who also shared them, privately, with me. Thank you.

Patient Stories

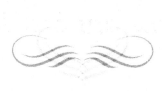

Russ

It's a Wonderful Life

In 1996, at age 34, I crossed the finish line of my first 10k race. I was in good physical shape and felt like I could conquer the world. In fact, I had just finished my graduate education and planned to move to Germany and put my Masters Degree in International Trade to good use. Two months later I was being treated for a persistent cough that had been diagnosed as bronchitis.

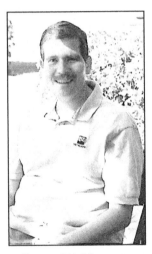

Russ and his Heartmate

Only the cough did not get better, instead it became much worse until I ended up at St. Joseph's Hospital in the emergency room. I am alive today because the doctors in the emergency room did an echocardiogram, which showed that I had cardiomyopathy. I was told that the only treatment was a heart transplant and was referred to the University of Michigan Medical Center.

Over the course of the next two years with diet limitations and medications I was able to hold my own. It's funny thinking back that I felt pretty good but I was not able to run 10k races anymore. Approximately two years after being diagnosed my world started getting smaller and smaller thanks to heart failure.

It became harder to sleep flat on my back and I ended up sleeping propped up on pillows. I noticed that a simple walk to the car was getting more difficult. When the drugs stopped working, I was admitted to the University of Michigan Hospital. There I was fortunate enough to come under the care of Dr. Pagani and Dr. Nicklas. Initially, I spent two months in the hospital. A new device was in clinical trials and I was one of the lucky recipients of the Vented Electric Left Ventricular Assist Device (Heartmate VE).

This device helped save my life. My heart had deteriorated so rapidly that I was not getting adequate oxygen to my brain. I remember hallucinations and crazy behavior in the hospital, but also losing track of days before and immediately after the surgery.

One day about a week after my surgery, a red haired woman came into my room and sat down and started talking to me. I tried to be polite and understanding but finally I had to ask her who she was. I was astounded to find out that this person was Ruth Halben, the social worker and she told me that this was the 3rd time she'd introduced herself! I didn't forget her after that.

I started to feel pretty good relatively quickly, started to walk the halls for exercise and even had some friends bring in my computer and started working a few hours every day while still in the hospital. On one of my walks I dropped in on another LVAD recipient in his room and sat down on a low stool. We were talking for a while and then finally we heard over the PA, 'will Russ please return to his room' ... well, I found that I couldn't get up! We finally figured out that if my friend pressed his call button, the nurse would come and help.

After about a month on the HeartMate the FDA announced that the HeartMate VE had passed the trials and would be approved. I was asked if it was OK if they took some video and photos of me for the news release and a photographer and videographer came out. They did a professional interview and we went out to the Botanical Gardens for a few photos. It was good to get out of the hospital. Afterwards I was told that the video was shown on

I will be eternally grateful for these volunteers who showed up faithfully and reliably week after week.

2

the national evening news and about 6 million people saw it ... I guess that was my 15 'seconds of fame.'

My friends and family and this new device made it possible for me to go home. I was one of the first allowed to go home on the LVAD and at that time the doctors wouldn't let me go unless someone was going to be with me all the time. There was a 30 to 45-minute training session that anyone who was to be with me needed to go through in order to learn what to do in different scenarios including how to change batteries and manually pump the Heartmate.

The president of my church council offered to organize the volunteers and we had several training sessions in the waiting room at the hospital for a total of 29 volunteers. I went home in mid-September and every week my wife and I would sit down with the church president to determine the times we needed coverage for "Russ Sitters." I will be eternally grateful for these volunteers who showed up faithfully and reliably week after week.

The weekend before Thanksgiving one of the valves stuck open on the HeartMate and I was re-admitted to the hospital. After much discussion, the doctors decided not to replace the device, but rather to wait until a heart was available because it seemed to be functioning adequately and having another surgery would take me off the active transplant list for a few weeks.

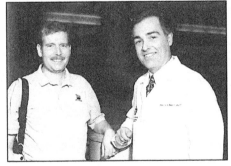

I felt so good even with a malfunctioning pump that I wasn't sure I wanted a heart transplant. Dr. Pagani told me repeatedly that they've never had a December without a transplant ... as I waited impatiently in the hospital.

Russ with Dr. Pagani

On January 1, 1999, I received my precious heart. I feel truly blessed to have received a chance to live this wonderful life. It has made me aware of all the supportive friends and family that reached out and touched my life in such

3

positive ways. It has helped me appreciate the present and be thankful for what I have in my life.

I continue to work full-time, have a sweet and intelligent daughter who was born after my transplant, new experiences and many opportunities to give back to my community. I am one of the select few that can honestly say, "I left my heart" at the University of Michigan.

Risa

Heart to Heart

Twelve years is a long time — sometimes when I think back, I have to remind myself that it really happened. The scar that I see every day between my breasts is a reminder that at one point in my life, the beat of my heart depended on batteries and a mechanical device implanted in my chest.

I was exactly where I always thought I would be in life on the verge of turning thirty: the married mother of a beautiful two-year-old daughter with another little girl on the way. My days consisted of play dates and naptime, while I suffered from relentless nausea and fatigue. During the 23rd week of my pregnancy, I entered a local hospital for hydration and observation.

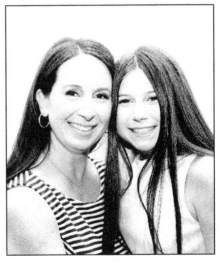

Risa and her daughter, Allison

I only planned to be away for the night; I could not imagine on that beautiful fall day that I would not return home until Christmas. It turns out that I had more than just morning sickness — I was in acute congestive heart failure due

5

to an atrial myxoma, a benign heart tumor that needed to be removed in order to save my life.

I was sent by helicopter to the University of Michigan Health System. By the time my family drove to Ann Arbor, I was being prepped and readied for surgery.

The surgeons succeeded in removing the tumor, but my heart continued to flounder, and I started to develop multi-system organ failure. While still unconscious, I delivered a stillborn little girl who weighed just more than a pound and who was unable to survive the trauma to my system. I was placed on an extracorporeal membrane oxygenation (ECMO) machine to bypass my heart and lungs. My family was given grim news — even if ECMO saved me from severe brain damage, I would need a new heart, but my body was too weak to survive transplant surgery.

To say I was lucky sounds strange and even a little farfetched, but if you need a new heart and your body is not strong enough to get one, having access to a left ventricular assist device (LVAD) is better than winning the Lotto. Between the tumor surgeries, stillbirth, and ECMO, my heart and body needed a rest. Even having an LVAD implanted was risky due to my weakened state.

When I finally regained consciousness four weeks after I had entered my local hospital, I found myself attached to a strange device plugged into the electrical outlet next to my bed. I heard loud sounds coming from the middle section of my body, and a wire was coming out of a hole in the side of my chest — a literal lifeline. My family and the doctors did their best to explain what had happened. They told me that I was on the heart transplant list and that the mechanical device ticking inside of me would enable me to go home while I waited for a donor organ.

Compassionate nurses taught my mom how to clean the opening for

> **To say I was lucky sounds strange and even a little farfetched, but if you need a new heart and your body is not strong enough to get one, having access to a left ventricular assist device (LVAD) is better than winning the Lotto.**

the driveline, a process that would become our bedtime ritual. Dressed in a full protective gown, she would have to keep the hole clean and free of infection. My doctors needed to know that my family could take care of me outside the confines of the hospital, so before I could be discharged, my father and I were required to spend a night in a hotel room connected by a long corridor to the main hospital. A medical supply company delivered supplies to my house. Finally, on Christmas Day, with a suitcase full of batteries and a holster on my back, I went home.

The main charging device sat on the nightstand next to my bed; the cord was just long enough for me to be able to go to the bathroom in the middle of the night without having to be disconnected. Every morning, I dressed in loose fitting clothes that were a few sizes too big. I could not wear anything tight around my middle section because I had to leave room for the driveline to stay covered and secure in place. The holster on my back held two fully charged batteries. Breakfast was served with many pills and a blood pressure check; I logged every reading in a diary that was reviewed during my visits to the doctor. I wore the holster all day, changing the batteries every six hours when the low power alarm beeped. There was no surprising anybody — you could definitely hear me coming.

I could never be left by myself; I always had to be with someone who was trained to take care of me. In order to build back my strength and to prepare for future surgery, my doctors encouraged me to exercise. Michigan winters are not conducive to outdoor activities in patients with heart failure, so my sister and I joined a local gym that had a walking track. We strolled together a few times each week, pulling my emergency suitcase of batteries and supplies on every journey. I did not move fast and it was exhausting, but I was glad to be out of the hospital and trying to regain my strength. This precious time with my sister was even more special because we both knew how close we had come to losing each other.

A patient hooked up to batteries with an electronic device in her chest cannot shower or be submerged in water. Lucky for me, I did more freezing than sweating in the frigid Michigan cold. I learned how to give myself a sponge bath, and I learned how to accept help from my loved ones who offered to

7

Those test days were some of the hardest I experienced throughout my entire ordeal. My LVAD was temporarily turned off and I was poked and prodded while my heart was taxed with chemicals and exercise.

assist. I went once a week to a local salon, where they washed and dried my long hair. One of the manicurists at the salon even bought separate tools to do my nails; I could not risk getting an infection from implements that had been used on others.

As I regained strength, I ventured out a little more. I visited close friends, and I went to the occasional restaurant for a meal. This was an emotional challenge. Many in my community were following my story and wanted to get a glimpse of me. Stories had spread that I had suffered horrible effects from my lengthy stay in the hospital, that I looked and sounded different, that I had somehow changed. I craved anonymity and I longed for the day when I could go about my life, living on my own, without people following my every move.

I trekked back and forth to the hospital on a regular basis. A nurse was assigned to accompany me to every visit and every test. I had her personal cellphone number, and I could call her at any time, day or night, with questions or concerns. At every return visit, I had the same question for my doctors — when could I be free of the wires? I was young, I had been in good health prior to my pregnancy, and I had no history of coronary heart disease. Within a month of my return home, the discussion had shifted from planning a heart transplant to the real possibility that my heart had healed enough to have the LVAD removed. This recovery was motivation for me to continue building back my strength; I was willing to do whatever the doctors told me to do.

In order for the LVAD to be removed without a transplant, I had to go through a series of tests so that the doctors could be certain that my heart was healthy enough to pump without assistance. Those test days were some of the hardest I experienced throughout my entire ordeal. My LVAD was temporarily turned off and I was poked and prodded while my heart was taxed with chemicals and exercise. All the while, I was shadowed by doctors and nurses who were ready at a moment's notice to re-connect my wires if needed. That stationary bicycle still gives me nightmares, but I knew I did not have a choice, and if I was going to regain my independence, this was something I had to do. One test even had to be repeated, just to be 100% certain I was ready. It turned out, I was.

Almost two months to the day after my discharge from the hospital and almost three months after the LVAD had been implanted; I entered the hospital to have the life-saving machine removed. I had been unconscious for all of my previous surgeries, but this time I was aware of what the surgeon was planning, and I was terrified. I was so grateful for my miraculous recovery, but I panicked at the thought of returning to the intensive care unit. I told myself that I had made it this far and there was no turning back. I remember being wheeled into the hallway on the way to the operating room, and then I woke back in the ICU as they took me off the ventilator. Aside from the pain down my chest, I felt well. There was a large hole in my side where the driveline had been removed. I vividly remember the beautiful silence; with the LVAD gone, there were no whirling or clicking noises.

After that final week in the hospital, I asked my doctor what came next. My life since that beautiful fall day had been consumed with survival and surgeries. My family and I had been forced to hope for someone else's tragedy in order for me to have the possibility of getting a new heart. We had prepared ourselves for a life with an LVAD, or maybe two or three LVADs, as some people need to have a new one implanted once the old one wears out. I had somehow beat the odds and survived. The doctor looked at me and told me to go home and live my life, so that is exactly what I did.

After the LVAD was removed, I went through six months of cardiac rehabilitation, and it was another six months before I fully regained my strength. I started to go out more, and people seemed to stare less. The hole in my side closed up just as they said it would, and my visits back to the hospital became more infrequent. Life slowly started to return to normal, or what I considered my "new" normal after such a life-changing event.

I used to think about my ordeal every single day; it was hard not to. I was so sick…and then I wasn't. I had joined a very small group of the population who can actually say that modern medical technology saved their life. Those trips

9

back to the hospital for follow-up tests and doctor visits eventually became less frequent. I now only see my cardiologist once a year, when we share stories about our families and pictures of our kids. Most of the hospital staff who knew my daughter when she was a toddler running through the halls of the hospital have a hard time believing that she is now in high school. I volunteer in the hospital every month; it makes me feel good to give back to a place that saved my life, and I hope that others can benefit as I share my story. I cannot explain why I developed a tumor or why I had such a miraculous recovery — I just know that I am very lucky and extremely thankful.

LVADs have shrunk over the past decade. When I talk about my experience with today's cardiac patients, I am reminded of trying to explain to my daughter what life was like without cellphones and the Internet. It makes me wonder how I survived. I am so grateful that an LVAD was available when I needed it. It was not just a bridge to what could have been a transplant; it was a passage to a second chance at life.

David

Pushing the Limits

My name is David. I am 75 years of age. My "heart story" began when I had a heart attack in 1982 at the age of 41. The left ventricle of my heart was damaged. In 1999, I had quadruple bypass. At the time, the surgeon told me that my heart was not in the greatest condition but all was fine for a couple of years. Then my heart began to worsen. Congestive heart failure set in. My heart was in bad shape and my cardiologist suggested going to the University of Michigan for a consultation. After several visits to a U of M cardiologist, I had an appointment with Dr. Pagani.

After the first meeting with Dr. Pagani, it was decided that my condition was not bad enough for surgery, so for a time I made periodic visits to U of M to keep an eye on the situation. The doctors talked about the heart transplant list. The congestive heart failure had progressed to the point that it was affecting my life.

I could no longer do everyday things. I could not even walk

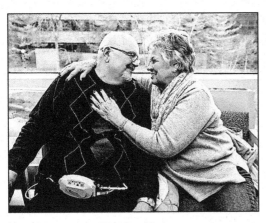

David and Judy

up ten stairs without having to stop and catch my breath. At that point, Dr. Pagani began to talk with me about a heart pump to help me until a new heart became available.

A new LVAD was in the experimental stages from Thoratec, the Heartmate II. Dr. Pagani talked to us at length and even drew a picture of it on the exam table paper at his old office in the Taubman Center. He showed my wife and I and two of our sons what it looked like and how it worked. For the four of us, it was an easy decision. We agreed that we should go ahead with this new pump. I was at ease with the direction we were going in.

Surgery took place on May 26th, 2004. I was the first patient at U of M to receive the Heartmate II and the second in the United States. After the LVAD was "installed," I felt 100% better. After 11 hours in a cool surgical suite, I had warm hands and feet. I also lost the grey pallor that I had. My wife commented that I finally had a warm feel. I was able to do everything that I had to stop doing before the LVAD was put in. I was able to ride my bike, walk and even go back to doing woodworking projects. Though this last hobby was curtailed when I ran my controller into a table saw blade, while it was running. Needless to say, this was not popular with Dr. Pagani and the LVAD staff.

My second year into life with the LVAD brought my only chance at a transplant. Unfortunately, the donor heart had started to deteriorate and it was decided not to use it. As far as it being the only chance at a transplant, it was determined that the anti-bodies in my blood were elevated and it became a difficult, if not impossible match. As time went on, it was eventually decided to take me off the transplant list. I would live the rest of my life as I was. Between the third and fourth years, I ended up with a driveline infection.

I was the first patient at U of M to receive the Heartmate II and the second in the United States. After the LVAD was "installed," I felt 100% better.

This would not clear up and eventually the LVAD was changed and the driveline site was moved. Approximately 18 months after the second LVAD was put in, I had another driveline infection. I was fixing the outside faucet under my deck and broke the seal

12

while lying on my stomach. There have been times when I pushed the limits of things that I should and should not be doing. As I mentioned previously, the Controller and the saw blade had their chance meeting and later, after my hand also ran into the same blade and cut off two fingers at the first knuckle, the law was laid down. My wife said no more.

Three months after cutting off my fingers, I fell down the stairs of our deck and suffered a compound fracture of my ankle. The foot was broken clean off the ankle. Because of my diabetes, they were unable to cast it. I was placed in an immobilizer, hoping the open fracture would heal. It did not. After suffering through three months of the most intense pain I've ever felt, I had a below the knee amputation of my left leg. I have a prosthesis and am getting along fairly well with it to date.

On May 26th, 2016, I will have had my LVAD for 12 years. I am the longest living person on the Heartmate II. This has been a family affair. My wife does not have a nursing degree but over the years she has become very proficient in taking care of my needs. She is an outstanding caregiver.

My family and I will be forever grateful to the University Hospital, the Circulatory Assist Clinic, the LVAD coordinators and all of the doctors I have seen through the years, especially Dr. Pagani. Without him and his staff, I would not be here today. I would not have seen my four granddaughters grow up and I would not be writing this today. The whole experience has changed our lives for the better. Thank you again and God Bless you all.

Chuck

Heart 2 + LVAD 1 & 2

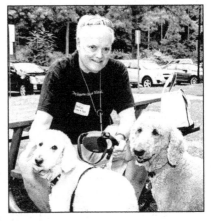

Chuck with Tess & Rusty

Chuck in the year 2000 was a 57-year-old white male with no significant health issues. I noticed while walking uphill to work that I became out of breath. Not unusual and I just thought that I was "out of shape," to use my lay terminology.

My wife, Tracey, an M.D. Pathologist at St. Joseph Hospital noticed a change in my behavior including lethargy, general lack of energy, shortness of breath, and a cough. She insisted that I make an appointment with a pulmonologist, who thought I had asthma. I was treated for asthma, but continued to get worse. After a few months, a family friend, then a cardiologist at the Michigan Heart and Vascular Institute (MHVI) agreed to introduce me to a colleague who took me on as a patient. A heart catheterization then showed that I had severe heart failure, but with clean arteries. The husband of one of Tracey's partners was a vascular surgeon, and he took a look at my heart cath films and said, "Chuck, you have a problem." That got my attention, coming from a friend who did not mince words.

With medical treatment I got a lot better, but then in the next few years my heart failure continued to progressively worsen. By the end of 2003, my cardiologist felt that I should be transferred to the University of Michigan Heart Failure Program, as there was nothing more, medically, that

I drive two wonderful Therapy dogs to their jobs every week where we try to give back as much as we can to bring a smile to patients and staff we knew while I was a patient at the UM hospital.

could be done for me. By this time, I had a pacemaker and an onboard defibrillator just under the skin of my left chest muscle.

In 2003 and 2004, my heart failure became worse, to say the least, and the good people at UMHS ordered a battery of tests followed by a consultation with a noted heart surgeon and a social worker. It seemed we talked only briefly before I was asked if I would like to have a heart transplant. There was a serious explanation of the risks involved, and it took no time at all for me to say YES right then and there. I had a young family and wanted to see them grow up. By the fall of 2004, I couldn't climb the stairs to our sleeping floor and it was difficult to walk the dogs around the block. Finally, it was tough to walk to the bathroom.

After more tests verified that my other solid organs were in OK condition, I was given an Assist Device (LVAD) with two external batteries and tubes into and out of my chest and attached to my heart to help circulate blood to the rest of my body, most importantly to my brain where I showed signs of forgetfulness. I felt much better immediately after the surgery, and went home after seven weeks in the hospital where I was impressed by the quality of care that I received by the entire staff, especially the nurses who insisted on taking vitals every so often. They had to "gown up" when cleaning my wounds and changing the dressings. The objective was a sterile field. Infection would be a bad thing.

After 13 months my first LVAD became worn out and another LVAD, a Heart Mate II, was installed in the fall of 2005. It was improved by being smaller and it was quiet. It was a small price to pay for another year of family and friends.

Some friends came to my room to play bridge and poker. Apparently this was a first. I did what I was told and even took most of the pills provided every four hours. Some of those pills were to counter the side effects of other pills. I was a good patient, but I could not remember to ask the surgeon questions from day to day until a list was made for me to use.

In June of 2006, I was called at 4:10 am to ask how long it would take me to get to the hospital. They thought a heart was available that met my profile, after two years of waiting. We were to arrive about 5:30 am, which allowed me time to send an email to the kids, my brother and several friends to tell them what was happening. I later learned that I was a bit casual about it on the phone, but the kids and brother from Traverse City arrived by about noon to wish me luck. By 3:00 pm all conditions were a go, so I was rolled down to the OR where there appeared to be about twelve people there waiting for the main event. Apparently, it took me a day to wake up and face the news that all went well. Twelve days later I went home with my new heart and the start of my new life.

After twelve months at home, I was presented with an infection in my breastbone. It took only a few days to determine what infection it was and how to treat it. So I went for another surgery where my chest was cracked open for the fourth time since 2004 and the infected bone was removed. Staples were used to close the wound, and after healing I pleaded with my surgeon's nurse to take all forty-four of them out, knowing that she was a sympathetic soul and wouldn't hurt me too much.

Now nine years post-op, I am back to health according to my cardiologist who sees me every six months for follow-up visits. Other than taking 17 pills per day for the rest of my life, I am fine. Thanks go out to my children and their spouses (two PharmD's, three MBA's, a high school counselor, and an environmentalist) and a very tired M.D. slash wife. I would say now and forever that I would not have been a good patient without them.

Nowadays my life is filled with sports I used to like such as golf. I also play bridge and poker, and help the referees and umpires with my season tickets at UM sporting events. I do volunteer work for a service club, and I drive two wonderful Therapy dogs to their jobs every week where we try to give back as much as we can to bring a smile to patients and staff we knew while I was a patient at the UM hospital. I have also traveled with my wife on group tours of Spain, the UK, and the Danube River, as well as a family trip to France. I still have not returned to a fixed schedule or a full-time job. I do, however, watch over the remodeling of our kitchen and two bathrooms. We don't intend to move until Tracey retires and gets involved in all the things she has on her very extensive list of "items to do when I retire."

S. Chand

My LVAD Saved My Life

I was born on June 2, 1943, at 9:35 am in a little town named Pasrur in India, now part of Pakistan. In 1947, my family migrated to New Delhi, India due to the political division of India and Pakistan, ruled by the British Empire. Being of Hindi religion, we had no choice but to come to India. My father was the Comptroller General for the Finance Ministry under Prime Minister Indira Gandhi for five years.

I obtained my Senior High School standing at age 15 years. I received scholarships for both Bachelor of Commerce and Master of Commerce Degrees from University of Agra, India. I went on to earn a Bachelor of Laws degree from University of Delhi, majoring in real estate and contract law.

I came to the United States from India in 1971 on a one-way ticket to New York with my final destination of Detroit. I had received a scholarship to attend University of Detroit and I achieved a Masters of Business Administration from there in 1972. My interest in finance was kindled by my father's success, expertise, and personal tutelage during my youth.

During this time, I worked as a dishwasher and bus boy for Normandie Bar & Grill in Detroit and used this money to help support my parents back home in

Coming to America, I planned to live the American Dream but health problems would delay that dream for a while.

India. While working as a kitchen helper, I met many wonderful people who contributed to my personal and financial growth. I saved $8000 and bought a duplex and started investing in real estate.

Coming to America, I planned to live the American Dream but health problems would delay that dream for a while. In September 2014, I faced heart failure with an ejection factor of 17%. My primary care physician Dr. Vijay Khanna, recommended I should see Dr. Francis Pagani, and gave me a tape of my heart performance to take to the appointment.

The visit was like a gift from God. I was impressed with his knowledge and was admitted for treatment and waiting for an LVAD to be implanted in my body to keep me alive. Ruth Halben, Dr. Aaronson, and Dr. Cho also welcomed me. I felt at home and hoped they would save my life.

My operation for LVAD was on December 8, 2004. I was able to leave the hospital on December 22, 2004. I am an entrepreneur and I was able to return to work on a limited basis. Part of my work is attending court on behalf of various business enterprises. On my first visit there, my LVAD equipment was a challenge for the security officers and electronic surveillance equipment but we got through it.

On February 17, 2005, I had my heart transplant. I am still living a perfect, healthy, normal life. I have expanded my education and exceeded every goal I have ever set for myself. I intend to continue to succeed. Thanks to the LVAD surgery, I am still living the American dream.

I hope the LVAD makes a difference in many people's lives as it did mine.

Ralph

A BiVAD Story

My story began in 2002 when I was diagnosed with atrial fibrillation. I was told this condition could cause dangerous blood clots and possibly a stroke. Doctors said that I would need a pacemaker. Two years later I had a pacemaker but one month after implantation I developed a dangerous irregular heartbeat known as ventricular fibrillation. I was rushed to the hospital and received an Implanted Cardio Defibrillator (ICD) that seemed to solve my problem.

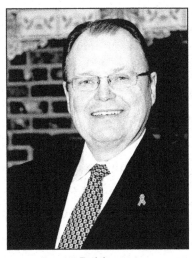
Ralph

Soon I was back to my normal routine of swimming six miles a week but that all changed in February of 2005 when I got a sinus infection. I received an antibiotic that had a negative interaction with Coumadin, a blood thinner, which caused blood clots. The pulmonary embolism or clot in my lung compromised the right ventricle in my heart.

After a month in the hospital and the placement of a Greenfield filter to preclude any other blood clots migrating to my lungs or heart I was transferred to the University of Michigan Hospital to be evaluated for a heart transplant.

The doctors decided that the clot would eventually dissolve and I would recover. I languished for two weeks unable to regain any stamina. Two trips to the hospital did not help pinpoint the continuing problem. The last trip to the emergency room had me being fast-tracked for a heart transplant. Unfortunately, soon after this decision my right ventricle completely failed.

The only thing that could bridge me to a heart transplant was a BiVAD (both right and left ventricular assist device). My heart was dysfunctional and my lungs soon failed. They could not do the BiVAD surgery. The U of M medical team, led by Dr. Haft, put me on an external heart and lung bypass machine known as ECMO (Extracorporeal Membrane Oxygenator). Simply put this machine pumped the blood for my heart and oxygenated the blood for my lungs so my lungs could rest and repair themselves. My family was offered a small chance of success of making it to BiVad surgery. Several days later my kidneys failed and dialysis was started. After ten days on ECMO, the medical team, with Dr. Haft leading the way, decided to surgically implant the BiVAD. However, shortly after surgery my lungs went into complete failure. I was to remain on a ventilator for months. My kidneys remained in total failure and my liver took a downward spiral into failure.

It was the 4th of July; I had been sedated since the middle of June and would continue to be sedated until mid-August. The surgical scar on my chest would be well healed before my eyes would open again. All told, my stay in the intensive care unit (ICU) would be three months. Nurses were kept busy with a myriad of equipment. Doctors poured over an ever-growing log of medications and collected data. My wife watched me struggle every day to gain a foothold on life. A staph infection invaded my bloodstream. A deadly bacterium was cultured from a needle tip. Things were looking dire. The doctors had

I am blessed. Most people with multiple organ failure don't survive. I recovered well beyond expectations. So well that within six months I was back in the pool swimming 100 laps three days a week.

discussions in hushed tones. They wanted me awake and let them know where we all stood. Sedation was slowly lifted and I became aware. I offered them my thumbs up.

A regimen of antibiotics was flooded into my body to defeat the infections. A body whose muscles had atrophied and was dependent on a ventilator and dialysis. I spent weeks with physical therapists just to get out of bed and on my feet. It was no picnic to learn to walk again. A tracheostomy allowed for a slow weaning from the ventilator. My kidneys slowly improved with improved blood flow from the BiVAD. Therapy helped me learn how to eat foods again after the feeding tube was removed.

I left the ICU mid-September and spent the next two and half months in the step down unit of 4C. I continued all my therapies. I worked up to walking a mile a day in the halls of the hospital. It was a lot of hard work but each day I felt I was getting closer to going home to waiting for the gift of life.

On November 30th, I achieved enough body strength and mobility that I went home. It was a great feeling to finally go home after six months in the hospital. It was scary to be away from the hospital but after a few days that feeling went away. My wife and I went shopping, out to movies and dinner with the BiVAD. The restaurants and movie theatre were very accommodating to seat us near an electrical outlet. Theaters have electrical outlets near handicapped seating. You see, my BiVad compressor was the size of a small rolling suitcase, needed to be plugged in most of the time. There was only a small window of time to run on batteries. It was great to spend Christmas and New Year's Day with my family.

I was back at the University of Michigan Hospital on January 15th because the compressor on my BiVAD was malfunctioning. Dr. Haft said, "You are staying in the hospital until a heart is available." Three weeks later on February 11th (my second birthday), I had my heart transplant and received my Gift of Life. Two weeks after the transplant, I went home, a new man.

I am blessed. Most people with multiple organ failure don't survive. I recovered well beyond expectations. So well that within six months I was back in the pool swimming 100 laps three days a week. In 2008, I participated in the Transplant Games and won multiple gold medals swimming. My quality of life is good.

I would not be here to today if not for God, my wife and all of the doctors, nurses, and trained staff that gave me the best of their talents at the University of Michigan Hospital during my long recovery. Special thanks to Dr. Haft, who recognized that I had the will and determination to make this a successful journey. The University of Michigan Cardiovascular Center truly made my Michigan Difference.

Wynonia

Our Sister JoeAnn & the LVAD

JoeAnn began utilizing the LVAD system after a string of heart attacks that began in the late 1990s. JoeAnn adjusted to the system very well as she was able to participate in most of her everyday activities such as bathing, showering and her appearance. JoeAnn did make an adjustment in regard to her clothing — using the device caused at least one change as she had to acquire and wear clothing that either fit over the device or under it.

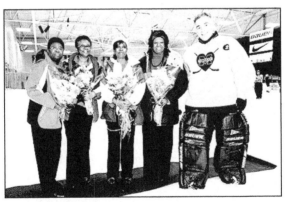

L to R: Wynonia, Yvette, JoeAnn, Kasandra and JoeAnn's cardiac surgeon, Dr. Francis D. Pagani on the occasion of the sisters' beautifully executed acapella performance of the Star Spangled Banner at the 12th Annual Hearts on Ice Hockey Challenge, a fundraising benefit for patients of the Center for Circulatory Support at the University of Michigan Medical Center.

She did find that she was unable to wear full-length dresses; aside from this fact, she continued to be the "fashion model" she always was.

The device never hampered JoeAnn from attending events, participating in activities that required minimal physical engagement or going on trips. JoeAnn was always an active individual and she never really slowed down after becoming an LVAD recipient. It was nothing for her to get up early, get dressed, and go out of town, to the park, to the show, to a concert or any other event that she desired to take part in. She never complained that the device stopped her or made something impossible. To the contrary, she continually thanked God for enabling her to utilize the device to live a rich and full life.

The device allowed her to maintain all of the aspects of her life that were of utmost important to her particularly being able to engage in family functions, such as going to her nieces and nephews school events – she loved to attend her nephew's soccer games, her niece's basketball games, and her sisters' social events, which allowed her to bring family for dinners, auctions, award ceremonies and so forth.

JoeAnn was always thanking God and giving thanks to the people who made the LVAD device for allowing her to keep living and going forward. She would talk with anyone at any given time about her experience and how it didn't knock her out but helped to keep her uplifted and striving for a wholesome and enriched life.

Whenever she was at U of M hospital, and that was fairly frequent because of scheduled medical visits, she would volunteer to talk and share her experiences on the system with new LVAD patients and encourage them to see it as a positive and another tool in their tool kit to continue living a long and healthy life. We (her family) were always amazed and astonished at the things that she was able to do with the aid of the device. She amused us to no end with her upbeat and joyous attitude about life and living it to the fullest.

We (her sisters) were inadvertently blessed by her being on the device in that we were privileged to attend functions primarily out of town where she was asked to participate in giving her testimonial about using the device and how it helped her to live well and happy. She truly had positive thoughts about being on the device and used it well to live and enjoy her existence.

Needless to say, we were blessed to have had her in our lives after she received the device, for the many, many years that she lived with it. She was the matriarch of the family and kept us on our toes and moving forward in our lives.

Editor's note: JoAnn died after nine plus years living on one LVAD. She was a joy to work with, as were her sisters. It is with deepest gratitude that we share their story.

Siming

Crossing the Bridge

Bang! My husband and I felt a big jolt followed by screeching noises when we were waiting for the traffic light to turn green. We knew immediately that we were hit. When we stepped out of the car, we realized the rear end of our car was beyond repair. A few minutes later, we met a young man, nervous and shaking, who had just gotten his driver's license a month before.

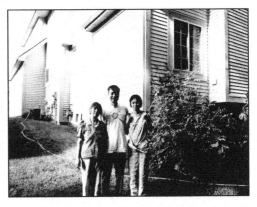

Siming with LVAD and her parents

This car accident didn't quench my excitement when I picked up my parents at the Detroit International Airport two days later. The last time I had seen them was one and a half years prior in 2004, when I visited them in China. This would be their first visit to Ann Arbor, MI. I had planned for them to stay with me for five months to enjoy the quiet and peaceful life in Ann Arbor. But I knew in just one week that they would accompany me through one of the milestones in my life.

The darkness

The spring had finally arrived in Ann Arbor after a long, cold winter. The sun was bright and warm. I proposed to my parents to walk to a nearby grocery store. A twenty-minute walk was not far. But on the way back home, I was out of breath. Walking on the flat walkway felt like climbing a steep mountain road. I sat down on the curbside to rest, unable to face my parents, because I knew what was in their eyes: concern, sadness, and helplessness toward their daughter.

On the coming Monday, I contacted the nurse who took care of congestive heart failure (CHF) patients. I complained to her about my worsened symptoms even though I had been following all the recommended rules for CHF patients including less water (I almost didn't drink any water even though I felt thirsty sometimes), less salt (no added salt to my cooking at all), and diuretic drugs. My BNP levels went up every time the doctor ran a blood test. My face was always pale. I was easily out of breath. I couldn't even raise my two hands above my head. I was distressed and scared of what might happen to me. Finally, on May 8th, after vomiting for no obvious reason, we decided to go to the emergency room at the University of Michigan Hospital.

The hospital ER was as busy as always. This was not the first time I had been to the ER; I knew I would be taken good care of once I was there. So I told my husband he could leave after I was admitted. I didn't want him to stay as he had just started his new job as a faculty member at the University. This was probably the most challenging time for him in his professional career. I had always felt guilty for bringing him so much trouble and taking him away from his work. One time, in an attempt to alleviate the guilt, I said to him, "If you just imagine you have a baby to take care, you would probably spend the same amount of energy and time at home not working." Deep in my heart, I knew there was no comparison between these two.

The moment I was wheeled into a single room in the ER, the nurses hooked me up to the IV lines, a heart monitor, and a pulse oximeter. Once connected, my room was like a supermarket, filled with all kinds of noise. The monitor would beep whenever my blood pressure dipped below 80. Unfortunately, my blood pressure was always below 80. So every time it measured, it beeped. Another noise came from a printer. Any irregular heartbeat would make the printer run. We would hear, "…da da da da…" every once in a while. And the paper strip just seemed to be spit out endlessly from the tiny printer.

Two doctors came in to check on me and asked, "What do you think might go wrong. You probably know better about yourself than we do." Encouraged by the trust, I said, "My symptoms are very similar to pericardial effusion which I experienced half year ago. And it was found out by echocardiogram. Could you check whether this is the case using echo?" Half an hour later, a big and heavy Echo machine was rolled in. I thought I could be a doctor myself after years of having heart disease. It turned out I was wrong. After contacting my cardiologist Dr. Aaronson, they decided to transfer me to the CICU (Cardiac Intensive Care Unit). I hoped that this hospitalization would be similar to my previous two stays. I would be sent back home after only a few days.

On the second day, I was pushed into an operation room for right heart cath. This procedure usually takes about one hour. A catheter is inserted through a neck vein directly into the right atrium and ventricle. The doctor can then take several important measurements of heart function, including cardiac output and pulmonary artery pressure. After the procedure, the catheter would still stay in there, to facilitate the administration of medications or to monitor heart functions. As I suspected, my cardiac output was only slightly above two, meaning approximately two liters of blood was pumped out of the heart per minute; the heart from a healthy individual is expected to pump four to five liters per minute. I also had high pulmonary pressure, which is common for heart failure patients.

Dr. Dyke, who is my age, was energetic and very considerate of his patients. I felt at home when I heard he would be my inpatient doctor. I'd met him about half year before when I was first admitted to the University of Michigan Hospital. He took the time to explain to me that patients with high pulmonary pressure were typically not suitable for heart transplant, because the new healthy heart never encountered pressures this high and would be unable to do well. As

31

a result, the right ventricle would have to work harder in order to pump the blood out. Patients would develop right heart failure and the survival rate was not good. To comfort me, he added that new medications were available to treat this condition and I would be put on those medications soon. In the meantime, I was quickly enlisted onto the heart transplant list as status 1A. There are a total of three major stages on the heart transplant list, status 1, 2 and 7. Status 1 can be further divided into 1A and 1B, with 1A being the most urgent where the patients need to stay in the hospital accepting medications to sustain his or her life.

Waiting always makes time pass by very slowly, whether you are waiting for your date to come, your food to be served, or waiting for the spring to arrive after a long, cold winter. The time trudges by even slower especially when you start to realize your hope is gradually sifting through your fingers. I was lucky to have my parents and my husband by my side every day. I was lucky to have support from friends all over the place. But these supports were slowly becoming too distant to hold onto. I felt like I was trapped on an island alone. Due to gradual loss of the appetite, I ate less and less and became so weak that I had to catch a breath in order to finish one simple sentence. So I spent most of the time not speaking at all. Every day, my parents just sat by the window next to me, not saying much either. Without looking into their eyes, I knew my mom was weeping and my dad worried about my worsening condition. Until one day I couldn't eat any more and started vomiting.

On that day, Dr. Dyke came in. When I looked at his face, I knew he had something to tell me. The medical intervention failed to lower my pulmonary pressure. There was only one choice left for me: the Left Ventricular Assistant Device (LVAD). Unfortunately, they were not sure if this was going to work because they had only observed in a few incidences when an LVAD device lowered pulmonary pressure. The LVAD is a mechanical pump that can be implanted into the chest. It is connected to the left ventricle to help the heart pump blood. The first generation of LVAD (Heartmate I), which had been approved by the FDA, was too big in size for me. The suitable model would be Heartmate II, which was smaller and remained in testing for clinical trials.

I had first heard of the LVAD about six months earlier. Three days after we moved from Boston to Ann Arbor. I had a cold and kept coughing every time I lied down. I could hear myself wheezing. I was so tired that I had to rest three times just to clean a small bathroom. My new primary care physician, Dr. Standiford, tried everything to help me feel better but to no avail. She arranged for me to have an echocardiogram. After the exam, I was urged by the technician to go to the University Hospital medical procedure unit immediately. Having gone through this kind of situation several times already, I was unbelievably calm. I asked my husband to drop me at the hospital main entrance. I then walked slowly to the medical unit on my own. I was admitted and rolled into the procedure room without too much of a wait. One hour later, the doctors told me I was experiencing pericardial effusion and they took out almost one liter of bloody fluid from the sac that surrounded my heart. Normally, the pericardium contains very little fluid. Under diseased conditions, fluid can build up and put excess pressure on the heart causing heart failure, or even death if untreated. Although I quickly recovered from this acute incident, I was still kept in the hospital while the doctors were working on figuring out what might have caused this.

One possible explanation for my pericardial effusion was that there might have been some defect with the lead of the defibrillator that I received several years before. The doctors proposed to remove the lead. Dr. Pagani, the head of the cardiothoracic surgeons, refused to perform this kind of open-heart surgery on a patient as weak as me and recommended LVAD at the same time. Maureen, Dr. Pagani's assistant, later explained to me in more detail about the LVAD. She even brought a LVAD pump to my bed to show me. However, I was still wondering what it looked like in a real person. So Maureen arranged a meeting for me. Although I couldn't remember his name, I still remember what happened on that day. He was wheeled into my room. He came to the hospital for a routine check-up. Unlike what I expected, his face had the glow of health. He was in such good spirits that it sounded so easy to live with an LVAD. I was almost convinced by him until I asked to see his surgical wound. When he slowly untied the gown, a long pink scar ran from his clavicle down to where the bandage was stabilizing the driveline. I held back my tears while continuing with more questions to cover up my emotion. I knew in my heart I was not ready for the LVAD, not at that moment, especially when I felt I could still get by without it.

It seemed to be my fate that I couldn't escape the LVAD. The difference this time was that I was ready, or more accurately, I had no choice. Many times, when I heard from friends and relatives saying I was brave, a cartoon would appear in my head. It is a man crossing a river by stepping on the heads of crocodiles. If you look behind him, you will understand why he is so brave: a tiger is chasing after him. *I had to become that man.* The surgery was initially scheduled for May 29th, twenty-one days after I was admitted to the hospital. The surgeon would be Dr. Pagani, who is one of the best heart surgeons in the country.

The first time I met Dr. Pagani was two days before the surgery; I had heard about him numerous times from other doctors, nurses and patients. He came in on his own; his hands in the pockets, and had a serious look on his face. I instantly felt a sense of trust toward this well-built, grey haired, middle-aged man. In a calm and low-pitched voice, he explained the procedure to me with only a few sentences, including how long it would take and other possible risks. Right before he left, he said, "This is going to be the most difficult thing in your life." To this day, that voice still echoes in my head every once in a while. Surprisingly, he returned to me five minutes later, "How about tomorrow?" "Fine with me, the earlier the better." I replied. It sounded like we had just rescheduled a dinner plan, not something that was going to be the most difficult experience in my life.

Although we didn't say much, I knew how my husband felt. After he went home, I sat on the bed digesting what Dr. Pagani had just said. The tears streamed down my face and I didn't wipe it. I knew I needed it to let out my fear, my worry, and the desperation deep in my heart. Right at that moment, Dr. Mordo stepped in to check on me and caught me weeping. He sat down by my bed and asked softly if it would be OK for him to talk to me. I knew Dr. Mordo from his daily visits. He was young and warm. His eyes told me I could trust him, or even rest my head on his shoulder if I needed. I grew up in a traditional Chinese culture where feelings for fear and love do not normally get expressed openly. But deep in my heart I needed to know. So I asked: "What kind of death is painful?" Maybe it is not unusual to chat about this in the CICU at all. He talked in a very calm and light-hearted tone. What I couldn't believe was that at the end we both started to make jokes.

After Dr. Mordo left, I had been thinking back and forth about whether I should leave a letter to my husband and my parents, telling them I loved them and thanked them for everything they did for me, in case I didn't wake up again. Eventually I didn't do it. I became too emotional to write anything the moment I picked up the pen and paper. Surprisingly, I had this belief that I would see them again.

The surgery
What happened on May 28th and the few days after was a total blur to me. I didn't even remember how I was pushed into the operation room; let alone how I came out of the OR.

But I did remember some conversations. Someone wanted to see me. The nurse told the person, "There is nothing to see. Her chest is open." However, that someone still insisted. The nurse probably reluctantly opened the door. "Ah!!!!!" Then I heard no more. Maybe he was so scared that he left the room. I also remembered, at one point, I heard a voice firmly say, "We have to take it out. It doesn't work!" It was this sentence that made me believe that I was going to die on the OR table because Heartmate II wasn't working. I then spoke to myself, or even tried to tell them, "Please let me go. I will donate everything." Later I curiously asked my husband whether any of these things actually happened, whether he ever insisted on seeing me. His answer led me to think that whatever I "heard" was probably from hallucinations due to the heavy usage of morphine. But those voices were so real that when I finally woke up from the surgery, I thought something else, other than Heartmate II, was implanted in my chest and saved my life.

They were scared by what they saw and didn't know what to do. One of the nurses said, "She still has her hands" meaning my hands were free of needles and they could hold my hands.

I didn't know how many days had passed before I opened my eyes. I found the room I stayed in was very noisy, vacuum sucking, machines beeping, people talking and walking, and so on. I tried to figure out the dates and pieced things together. But I certainly experienced some difficulties here, because I couldn't even remember when I had the surgery. For some reason, I believed the current time was sometime in July.

There were two nurses working around the clock monitoring my vitals, administering the medications, taking blood samples, responding to emergencies. On that day, I heard Mary, who was very experienced and skillful, was teaching Josephine. She instructed Josephine to try something. But I waited and waited, nothing happened. I almost wanted to turn around and tell Josephine, "Go ahead, I can take it." But I couldn't control my head at all. My neck was powerless. And I couldn't talk either because I was still connected to the breathing machine. I was totally dependent on this equipment and that was exactly what they were working on: to wean me off from the machine. The longer I was connected to the machine, the more difficult to wean off from it. I didn't understand what they were trying to do. All I felt was that Josephine was probably too scared to do anything. Finally, Mary was back in control, she quickly finished what they were supposed to do. Very soon, it was time for a shift change.

Surprisingly, Josephine asked if Mary was willing to stay and continue to teach her. "No," Mary said. Then I heard them arguing outside and eventually Josephine won. Mary agreed to stay one more shift to teach her. I later heard from other people that Mary and Josephine were classmates in the nursing school in Malaysia. Josephine was so determined and eager to learn that she stayed another twelve hours. Eventually, her hard work paid off. She transformed from a nervous nurse, who seldom looked at me when she stepped into the room, to a confident, experienced, warm person. Five months later when I stayed over at TICU for heart transplant, she was all by herself taking care of patients.

Later that day, my parents and my husband came to visit me. I saw bright smiles that I hadn't seen for a long time on their faces. In those wrinkles, I found great relief from days of uneasiness and anxiety. Surprisingly, I didn't smile back. My brain was still affected by the horrifying images in my hallucinations and I was angry with them for making me suffer through so much pain, just because they didn't let me leave this world on the operation table. I couldn't talk, so I just stared at them. My husband Jiandie gently grabbed my hand into his hands. It was at that moment that I realized that I was having a fever. Or more accurately, I believed this would be my new normal body temperature for the rest of my life.

I was in this confused mental status for another two days before I was finally disconnected from the breathing machine. But I still wasn't able to talk. To help me to communicate with other people, Jiandie wrote down the 26 English letters on a paperboard, so I could point to the letters. Finally, I knew what was going on while I was sleeping or unconscious.

It was only four days, not a month, during which I was unconscious. On the day of the operation, both Jiandie and my parents went through an emotional roller coaster. To catch me before the operation, they came to the hospital at 6:00 am and were hoping to send me to the OR. The CICU was located on the 7th floor, while the OR was downstairs in the basement. So we had to use the elevator. Unfortunately, the elevator was full with just my bed. Therefore, they had to take another elevator downstairs. But when they came down, I was not in the hallway any more. Jiandie felt regret that he wasn't able say goodbye to me before the procedure. He later drove my parents back home to rest and stayed at the hospital all by himself. For him, the clock must have been ticking extremely slowly on that day. He is a person of action. Waiting is not what he is good at.

It was not until 4:00 pm that I was finally pushed out of the OR. Contrary to what I thought, the LVAD was successfully implanted into my abdomen. Once I was moved into the Thoracic Intensive Care Unit (TICU), two highly experienced nurses quickly connected me to all sorts of tubes and lines of more than twenty different medications. They constantly measured my blood pressure, glucose level, and kept adjusting the breathing machine. When my parents and Jiandie came in, they were scared by what they saw and didn't know what to do. One of the nurses said, "She still has her hands" meaning my hands were free of needles and they could hold my hands.

What was unexpected was I was rolled back into the OR two hours later. With the help of the LVAD my blood pumping function was significantly improved. Unfortunately, instead of getting 90~100% blood oxygen level, mine was only 50%. Jiandie and my parents were so worried that I would suffer permanent brain damage. It turned out that there was a hole between the left and the right ventricles. When the left ventricle did not work properly, this hole was not a big problem. However, when it became a powerhouse with the assistance from the LVAD, the blood in the right ventricle flooded into the left through that tiny hole. The blood, that was supposed to go to the lung to get oxygenated, was now pumped back to the circulation.

It was already past 10:00 pm when I was sent back to the TICU. Dr. Pagani waited in the room and didn't leave until my condition stabilized.

Recovery

To a person who had been saved from the brink of death, recovery seemed like a never-ending process. Every day I was dealing with new issues. Just when I was able to breathe on my own without a breathing machine, I started to experience diarrhea, which was soon followed by a urinary tract infection. All at the same time, the doctors and nurses were helping me to battle against kidney failure and acute pancreatitis. I was so caught up with these complications and many discomforts that I didn't even realize my face was not pale any more for the first time in many years.

With the help of painkillers, I actually didn't feel much pain at the incision on my chest. However, what I didn't prepare for was sleep deprivation. Thanks to the painkiller, every time I closed my eyes, I "saw" colorful objects flying by, from geometric patterns to mountain-lake scenic views. At the beginning I was so excited and tried to remember every bit of detail of what I saw. I thought of drawing these images once I got out of the hospital and naming them "the Art of Life." But gradually, these beautiful images turned into nightmares. One try after another, no matter how hard I tried to push them away, they kept coming back over and over again. I tried all kinds of sleeping aids, but nothing seemed to help. Although I was lying in bed 24 hours a day, the noise and the endless slide shows in my head kept me awake for almost six days.

Without sleep, a normal day felt like anywhere between 48 hours and 72 hours, especially with the bedridden restriction and various kinds of discomfort. One night, I asked my night-shift nurse Chris for another sleeping pill. He recommended Benadryl and I remembered one of my friends had also used it before. So I said, "Let's give it a try." I can imagine he must have regretted his suggestion. After the pills went into my blood stream, I kept sweating and got really wet. So I called in Chris and asked if he could find a towel for me. Of course, I couldn't do the drying myself. It was he who did the job.

Unfortunately, a few minutes later, I was wet and very uncomfortable again. In the meantime, I felt I was full of energy. I thought I didn't need to bother him if I could dry myself by sitting up. To my surprise, I actually did it by holding onto the bed rail. While I was so happy for myself, as I couldn't even raise the head two days prior, Chris came in shock. He quickly settled me back to the supine position and begged me not to get up again, because I tangled all the lines connecting me. Later, no matter how many times I told myself, "sleep, sleeep, sleeeeeep," my body and legs just didn't listen at all. Chris finally begged me, "Honey, you need sleep. Your brain needs rest." "I know, I know," I said. Now I truly understand the agony of not being able to sleep. My legs involuntarily kept moving and trembling. It was not until 8:00 am in the morning when Dr. Pagani did his morning rounds and prescribed me a dose of a sedative that I was able to finally close my eyes and had a really nice sleep.

Dr. Pagani, called the "Big Guy" by the nurses, with an air of authority, is highly respected by both patients and the staff. I once heard from a friend's friend mentioning that working with Dr. Pagani was stressful, because he welded his work, patients and his own reputation together and couldn't accept failure or abandonment. People working with him always feel nervous and being pushed for better. However, being his patient means that you can trust him, because he will fight for you. From Bill's response, I could tell that the nurses were afraid of him, but at the same time, they looked up to him.

In the TICU, the nurses worked in 12-hour shifts and started their day at 7:00 am or 7:00 pm. One morning, it was Bill's shift. The moment he came to my room, he started to arrange the IV lines and told me he had already studied my medication last night knowing what to do. About half way through, he realized he needed to get my vital signs right away for the doctor rounding. He rushed to finish the measurements. Just as he finished, Dr. Pagani came in. The moment Dr. Pagani left, Bill was out of sight too. When I looked for him, the other nurse said he was having breakfast. I laughed when I heard that. I didn't expect Bill to be that nervous.

Even though I knew I could put my life in his hands, I felt unable to be close to this stone-faced doctor and was as nervous as those nurses every time I saw him. As an experienced surgeon, Dr. Pagani always rounded the room with several other residents or students. His look was serious, and he seemed frugal on words when talking to patients. However, it was these daily visits that finally registered his warmth and humor into my heart. Eventually one day I asked him why he was always that serious. His answer made everyone laugh, "Because my face grows that way."

My condition was eventually stabilized after about a week in the TICU. I was then transferred to a regular single room, which was very quiet. I was happy to find peace there until I realized the pump, which was connected to the chest tubes sucking out fluid, was constantly roaring. I believed this also annoyed Dr. Pagani. He turned it off before I could even open my mouth to tell him. He then tried to persuade me to eat more, so my wound could heal faster. Although Heartmate II was smaller, it was still too big for a 90-lb person. Once the pump was put in, my stomach was squeezed to the side that I easily felt full after just a few bites. So I argued back, "I tried very hard to eat, and I am so full that the food is right at my throat now." He said, "Then swallow it!" We both laughed.

...working with Dr. Pagani was stressful, because he welded his work, patients and his own reputation together and couldn't accept failure or abandonment ... However, being his patient means that you can trust him, because he will fight for you.

To quickly recover from the surgery, getting my feet down to the floor was as important as taking medications. After I was moved to the regular room, Talat and Linsey, two occupational therapists, came to help me. Being able to walk again must be a very exciting experience for many patients, or

40

so I thought. However, I felt nervous, because this time I was not walking alone. I had to carry four things with me all the time: the pump (in my chest already), the controller (a small computer that controls the pump speed), and two batteries. I am not talking about AA batteries here. The whole rig weighed about eight to nine pounds. Imagine carrying a nine-pound computer as a 90-lb person who hasn't walked for more than a month, you will get the picture.

The nurses had seen many people like me. Of course they wouldn't allow me to chicken out. They patiently helped me to prepare the walking package. A big belt was wrapped around my waist, so the controller could hang over the belt. Then the two batteries were each put in their bags and I would carry them like a backpack. Once the controller was disconnected from the wall power supply, I was able to take my first step. It felt like I hadn't walked for centuries, forgetting how to walk with my back straightened up. My father said, "Look up." I wanted to, but with stitches in my chest and controller next to my belly, I could only look down to the floor and use one hand to tightly hold onto the moving medication pole to maintain balance. I felt like a curved dumpling, plump and awkward, slowly sliding on the floor. Nevertheless, I was happy that I could finally wobble around.

To encourage me and show me how beautiful it was outside, Talat and Linsey wheeled me to the garden on the second day. It's a small garden, surrounded by several hospital buildings. This garden must have brought so much life to the doctors, nurses, and patients here at

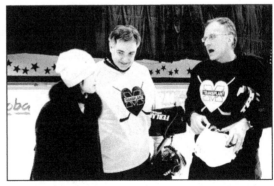

Siming with Drs. Pagani and Aaronson, geared up for hockey

the hospital. The moment we stepped out of the automatic door, my tears flooded in. I was speechless. The early summer of Ann Arbor was warm and wet. The bright sunlight made me squint. I took deep breath one after another, trying to sense every bit of the summer smell.

Inspired by this short outgoing, I set two goals for myself: exercise and eat. Gradually, I was able to walk three or four times a day. And every time I could walk a little bit farther. But eating seemed to be my biggest obstacle to full recovery. Dr. Pagani "threatened" me that they would insert a feeding tube if I still didn't eat much. I definitely didn't want another tube in and asked if I could eat the food my parents cooked. "Of course!" On the second day, a small fridge was moved into my room. So my parents could store some homemade Chinese food for me.

The number of the medications that went into my body through IV lines had greatly dropped and so did the chest tubes. I was so happy to see the light at end of the tunnel. And then I realized that being away from doctors and nurses was not as easy as I thought. I couldn't rely on them anymore and had to be on top of everything myself. There were about twenty different pills I was taking every day. For the past two weeks, the nurses had taken care of this. All I needed to do was to open my mouth when the little cup of pills was handed to me. Now I had to remember to take them and divide them into morning, noon, evening, and bedtime portions. With the LVAD pump, I needed to have my husband or my parents stay with me always. In addition to carrying a backup controller and batteries, we had to learn to judge emergency situations and know how to react. Although the controller is only as big as a CD player, it is much heavier. There are only two buttons and a few signal lights on the front panel. It looked simple, but with various combinations it can create many different signals. We had to know what kind of lights or noise means what. For example, a yellow light and long beep sound indicates the battery will be running out in 15 minutes; a red light suggests 5 minute of battery, the current batteries have to be replaced immediately, and so on. No matter how hard we practiced, it always seemed so complicated. It made me very anxious to hear any noise at all. Living on the pump was not as simple as it seemed.

The final training was for my husband Jiandie. The pump was connected to a controller through a dress line about one-third of an inch wide and 19 inches long. The line passed through the right abdominal wall. And a special material was used to wrap around the line to help the fusion between the body wall and the tubing. The merging of these two would take a very long time. If any infection happened at the exit site, it could have been life threatening. The area near the dress line needed to be washed twice daily. The procedure of washing was not difficult, though some basic sterile operation was required. The person needed to wear a disposable gown, a mask and put on surgical gloves. Everything in contact with that area needed to be sterile too, including surgical sponges and saline. To keep this area clean, I set a personal record by not bathing or showering for nearly half a year. Jiandie is a scientist doing biomedical research. His hands are as nimble as a surgeon's. But he hates doing any procedure on humans. For me, without hesitation, he trained himself to be my super nurse, putting on the appropriate gear to clean the dress line every day.

After we passed all of this training, I finally went back home three weeks after the surgery.

Back home

It was already summer. My parents told me they planted many vegetables in the garden. It was their dream to have a garden to grow things. I was very happy to see the backyard filled with greens. Ever since I was out of the hospital, my parents became my nutritionists and physical therapists. They tried to cook different food for me each day, so I could eat more to gain weight. We walked daily. If one day I got lazy and just wanted to rest, my father would drag me off the sofa and packed up things for me to go into the woods. At the beginning, I couldn't walk far carrying all my belongings. Occasionally I had to ask my father to carry the batteries for me for a little while. Gradually, I was able to climb up several hundred steps without taking a break.

Two weeks later I went back to see Dr. Pagani. Noticing the wound healing very well, Dr. Pagani decided to remove the stitches. The dense black threads, one by one, were cut and pulled out by him. About half way through, he noticed the room was really quiet and asked why I didn't say a word. "What do you want me to say? Scream?" I joked. Maureen, who had introduced the LVAD and had helped me tremendously throughout the process, grinned, "Some guys are much bigger than you. But they made noise." I smiled. I was actually holding my breath and taking this rare opportunity to observe this famous surgeon. He didn't have long bony fingers. Nor did he move swiftly as what I expected.

43

Instead, he was very slow and gentle. The more I got to know Dr. Pagani, the deeper respect I had for him.

It took me about three to four months to finally get used to this new life with the LVAD: carrying batteries and back up controller and batteries wherever I went; checking on the controller every half hour. I went back to work once things were stable. One good thing coming out the LVAD was that I finally could indulge myself with salty food. It seemed I had trouble maintaining body fluid. A certain amount of body fluid was required for a proper operation of the LVAD. So I was instructed to eat salty food, which I hadn't had much of ever since I started to experience the symptoms of congestive heart failure in 2004. I started enjoying life again, moving around without the need to pause to catch my breath. At one point I even thought I might as well stay on the LVAD for as long as possible even though I hadn't bathed for the longest time of my life.

As the "Bridge to Transplant," the LVAD successfully lowered my pulmonary pressure and got me physically and mentally ready for a heart transplant about four months later. I was enrolled back to the heart transplant list. On midnight of October 26, 2006, I received a phone call from the hospital, "I think we have a match for you." We packed up and headed to the hospital, and the next day, I received the most generous gift in my life: a new heart. That was the day that both the LVAD and defibrillator were removed from my body. That was the day my new life started.

One night not long ago, my one-and-a-half-year-old daughter rested her little head on my chest. Feeling the warmth of her tiny body in my arms, I whispered, "Baby, you are listening to mommy's heartbeat." My eyes were wet. For this moment, I have fought along with my family and friends. I owe a debt of gratitude to a dedicated medical team, from thoracic surgeons, cardiologists, nurses, social workers, administrators, technicians, to people who worked behind the scene. To my donor and donor family, I hope to continue a dream that they had started.

Edward

Active Retirement

G od, acting through Dr. Pagani and his team, has given many families the gift of life. We are just one family of many. In spring 2007 I had a serious heart attack. It was so serious that there was no sure solution unless I could get either a heart transplant or an LVAD. Almost 10 years later the LVAD was and is the gift of life for me.

During a right heart catheterization at the Toledo Hospital, I had my big attack. A balloon pump was attached to me and I was driven by emergency vehicle to University of Michigan Hospital where they might be able to do something for me. It was there that a few days later, Dr. Pagani and his team implanted the LVAD.

I was in the hospital for about seven weeks. Afterward, for about two years, my wife and I lived with my oldest daughter and her son and daughter because we needed the help with the recommended 24-hour supervision.

The LVAD treatment for me was truly a gift of life. When I first came to Michigan, I believed that my expected life was only a few days, so bad was my heart damaged. Here it is almost 10 years later and I lead a very active life.

Since 2007 my first great grandchild was born. My oldest daughter remarried. Now I have three great grandchildren. During this time one of my granddaughters and my brother died.

I am 79 years old and in, what I call, active retirement. I'm teaching four sections of astronomy at one college. Each semester, my teaching mix changes as I volunteer to teach classes that need to be taught but that many faculty don't want to teach. These are college level classes in astronomy, physics, statistics, mathematics, meteorology, physical science, and computer science. I have been paid by a publisher to evaluate new texts in statistics. I am writing a data analytics text with a table of contents and most of three chapters complete. My wife and I have made several presentations to college nursing students about my LVAD. For several years I have driven, often in a single day, to Atlanta, Georgia from Toledo, Ohio, doing it in reverse, a week or two later.

All of the above and more have been possible as a result of having an LVAD. The University of Michigan also maintains my LVAD. They not only saved my life but also improved its quality.

Those persons recruited by Dr. Pagani include nurses, aides, other physicians, social workers, and technicians — all are outstanding.

Marvin

A New Start

Ruth,

I could have written a book on specific events, and named the many professionals who worked to give me a wonderful "after-life (post-LVAD)." As I wrote that, and rewrote it many times, a lot of happy "memory tears" were shed.

Thank you. May God bless you.
Marvin

I was 49 when I experienced a "mild" heart attack. The resulting hospital stay and stent left me feeling much better and also more aware of my mortality. During the next twenty years there were more issues that resulted in a pacemaker, ablation, defibrillator, enlarged heart diagnosis, and many more hospital visits. I was slowing down internally and externally.

I was in the hospital again for heart issues. When my cardiologist entered my room, he shut the door. That was not his usual action, and neither was his serious expression. Lillian and I were holding hands as he explained there was nothing more he could do for us. He advised me to get hospice involved. I told him that his efforts had kept me going for 24 years and we thanked him for his expertise.

He wisely contacted a University of Michigan cardiologist, which, to me, really demonstrated his wisdom. When I entered the hospital there, a lot of interviews and more tests were more than I could have imagined but they determined that I was a candidate for an LVAD.

Every aspect of the procedure was explained, and after much prayer and total support from my family I opted to have the surgery. What a blessing that has been for the family and for myself!

I had given up all activities that involved physical exertion. I could not even stand up long enough to teach a Sunday school class. No fishing, no hiking, no hunting. The walk across the porch earned me a seat on the rocking chair. As I said before the quality of life was nearly non-existent.

I want to talk about how much this device has improved my life, but I cannot do that without praising the surgeons, doctors, and nurses who gave so much of themselves and their talents. I would be remiss not to mention the lady who became all these entities when I went home. She is my wife and my best friend.

What the LVAD has done for me…

I have resumed the joyful responsibility of teaching a Sunday school class. Can you imagine how thrilling it is to be able to do that again?

It is my job to mow between 4.5 and 5 acres of lawn at my son and daughter-in-law's home. Did I say job? I love the smell of newly mown grass.

Walking is no longer an issue. Twenty minutes on the treadmill has become a warm-up to a very active day.

I want to talk about how much this device has improved my life, but I cannot do that without praising the surgeons, doctors, and nurses who gave so much of themselves and their talents. I would be remiss not to mention the lady who became all these entities when I went home. She is my wife and my best friend.

Did I say active day? There are days I cut down dead trees and cut them into twenty-two inch logs. These must then be run through a log splitter so they can be fed into the outdoor boiler. Oh yes, I do that as well. Note: I wear shop coats to protect my controller and batteries.

I am able to hunt and fish…often successfully.

My wife and I travel. We stop frequently, not because of my LVAD, but merely observing proper protocol for a couple of seventy-something-year-olds who ought to take a walking break.

My family and I have been with this device since 2008. There have been many family events I would have missed without it: births, ballgames, graduations, birthdays, and reunions. Again, I would like to thank all those people involved with my health care.

Ruth,

If it weren't for you, Lillian would not have found a place we could afford so she could stay near me during my hospital stay. Please don't delete this accolade.

Thank you,
Marvin and Lillian

Michael

Pump Me Up!

Just because it isn't perfect, doesn't mean it isn't awesome. - M.R. Mathias

O ur lives are one entire story made up of individual smaller stories, a book with many chapters. Some of these stories may be thought to be 'interruptions' in the story of a life but in reality, they are part of that story. This is one of those stories in my life.

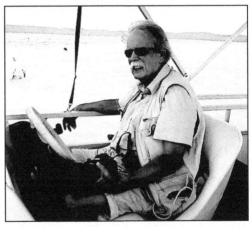

Mike on the Boat

Let me begin my story in December of 1982. I was 37 at the time. My father had passed away about a decade earlier at age 65. He unexpectedly collapsed at home just before going to work and died of a heart attack within twelve hours of being transported to the hospital by the EMS. My mother would, within a couple of years, pass away at age 59. She too unexpectedly collapsed at home after attending a wedding reception and died in the hospital of a heart attack, like my father, some twelve hours later. Neither

51

my father nor mother had any history of heart disease as both of their parents lived well into their eighties. Unfortunately, both of my parents were smokers, neither exercised and my mother was overweight, which may have contributed to their subsequent demise.

In December of 1982, I was in good health, having given up smoking seven years earlier, gone on a diet losing thirty pounds, and began an exercise program, jogging fifteen to twenty miles per week. I changed my eating habits to a lower fat diet and my blood cholesterol was at normal levels. I was looking forward to our annual ski trip with friends to Jackson Hole, Wyoming. Life was good and having changed my lifestyle, I presumed that any genetic predisposition to heart disease that I might have inherited would not significantly affect me.

I chose December of 1982 to begin this story as that was the month that a man named Barney Clark, age 61, made international news as the first patient to undergo surgery and receive a total mechanical heart. He had progressive heart failure and was not considered a candidate for a heart transplant because of concomitant health issues. I followed his medical course closely. As the first person to undergo this procedure he reportedly told his physicians he did not expect to live more than a few days, but in fact lived almost four months, 112 days. His quality of life, however, had much to be desired. His mentation was less than it had been before surgery with multiple episodes of loss of consciousness. His blood pressure often fell to low levels and he was plagued by multiple infections and blood clotting problems, which lead to several strokes. He became a hero for allowing himself to be the first person to have this procedure. I too considered him a hero and admired what he had done for the sake of scientific and medical progress, but did not consider the surgical procedure a success. His life may have been prolonged by several months but his quality of life seemed not improved; in fact, it deteriorated. It occurred to me the procedure could more accurately be described as prolonging his dying rather than increasing his longevity. I even believe it was reported that on at least one occasion he was asking to be allowed to die.

I had congestive heart failure. I had the same disease as Barney Clark and I was devastated; how could this happen to me? Just a few months earlier I was active and feeling well, but now I could hardly breathe and talk at the same time. Life was no longer "good."

I found it quite incomprehensible the ordeal Mr. Clark underwent. I had never really known another person with heart failure as severe as his and found it difficult to identify with his condition and situation. I did think of him as a hero and a rather brave man, but having followed his ordeal, thought to myself that under no circumstances would I allow any mechanical device to be placed into my body, or that it would ever become necessary.

I was healthy and feeling good. I was skiing in Jackson Hole, Wyoming and watching the Michael Jackson music video *Thriller*, a song he released about the same time as Mr. Clark had his artificial heart pump inserted. Little did I know that this music video might be the seed giving birth to the hit TV series *The Walking Dead* decades later. Little did I know that this remembrance of Barney Clark would haunt me in coming years when I too would develop severe heart failure and physicians recommend I have a mechanical device surgically implanted to assist my failing heart pump and circulate blood throughout my body.

Fast forward to the spring of 1998. Life was still "good." I was planning my next ski trip to Jackson Hole and had just returned from a two-week rafting trip along the Colorado River, through the entire Grand Canyon. The day before the start of the rafting trip with my wife and good friends, I jogged around the entire city of Flagstaff, Arizona. This would be the last time I would be able to really jog for a period of almost thirteen years. On the rafting trip we went on multiple long hikes and at the age of 53 I was looking forward to many more years of continued physical activity, skiing, camping and vacationing with my wife, two adult children and friends. This was not to be and my life was about to change.

After coming back to Michigan from this spectacular rafting trip, I developed a chronic cough with weakness that progressively became worse over the next few months. I was not able to jog more than a block or two without exhaustion and shortness of breath. I thought this might be due to a viral infection that would improve with rest and a tincture of time. When it did not improve, but worsened with a progressive loss of energy, persistent cough, weakness and difficulty climbing up one flight of stairs or even standing for any length of time without getting short of breath, I thought I might have pneumonia and should have a check-up. A chest x-ray was performed that revealed fluid on my lungs with an enlarged heart. I had congestive heart failure. I had the same disease as Barney Clark and I was devastated; how could this happen to me? Just a few months earlier I was active and feeling well, but now I could hardly breathe and talk at the same time. Life was no longer "good" and I was immediately admitted to the hospital Intensive Care Unit after a follow-up echocardiogram indicated advanced heart failure.

After I was hospitalized, a heart catheterization was performed the next day and drugs were given to help my heart pump better and control the excess fluid on my lungs. A diagnosis of congestive cardiomyopathy was confirmed and I was transferred to another hospital for consideration of a heart transplant. My mind was in a haze of what seemed like a surreal experience. While being worked up for a heart transplant, I was given water pills to keep fluid out of my lungs, and other drugs to aid my failing heart. I began to feel much better and improved to the extent that I was no longer considered ill enough to be a transplant candidate. I was, however, informed by the heart doctors that my heart disease was not curable, would progressively get worse with time, and I would likely be in need of a transplant within five years. I was subsequently discharged from the hospital, and with medication, able to do most normal activities without much shortness of breath, with increased energy and less weakness. I felt better than I had in months. I could no longer jog, however, or participate in any strenuous activity as I had in the past.

After discharge, I continued to feel even better with less shortness of breath and decided, after a period of time, that maybe the doctors were wrong and that I could have had a virus that affected my heart and with time would go away and so would my heart failure. This was wishful thinking, irrational, and a state of denial. With this denial or what I called optimism guiding my actions, I decided I was healed well enough to begin jogging again and maybe even able to ski in a year or so.

So, one morning I went outside to jog only to almost collapse after about 50 yards. Reality came crashing down on my optimism. A selfish anger then emerged from this change in my perception of reality. "This shouldn't have happened to me, what did I do to deserve this? After all, I quit smoking, lost weight, and exercised." I didn't deserve to have this happen but then, who was I to decide what I did or did not deserve and who was I to be angry at all? Despair and depression followed as I realized the doctors were right and I was wrong. For the first time, I was forced to face the fact that my disease was progressive and I was not going to get better, but even still I was hanging on to some sense of false optimism or denial. This was apparent when it was recommended that I have surgery to implant an ICD (Implantable Cardioverter Defibrillator) along with a pacemaker. I was told this device would give my heart an electrical shock if it began to beat with a rhythm that could stop my heart from pumping. I refused, still having an aversion to any mechanical type of device being placed in my body, and somehow thinking that this was not a necessary procedure for me at that time. I did not feel that sick but it's easy to deny a reality that you don't want.

I did reasonably well with medications and their adjustments until 2004 when I developed an emergent irregular heart rhythm and had two cardiac arrests in the Emergency Room of Beaumont Hospital. With this reality check, I consented to the placement of an ICD and pacemaker.

Living with the pump had become a new and rewarding experience in my journey with heart failure as the physical quality of my life had improved considerably. The memory of that first mechanical heart and Mr. Clark's 112 days faded along with my fear.

I had survived this near death experience very much aware that I'd lost consciousness two times. The experience affected me deeply. I remembered that we all die, even me, and a new sense of living and my own mortality now took center stage. Death comes to us all, something I knew but forgot and was now reminded of. This fresh knowledge of my own mortality gave me a newfound appreciation of my own existence apart from the rest of the physical world, in time and space, a gift not of my own choosing but of grace. I began to truly appreciate life and its many blessings, with the physical quality of life now being of secondary concern. I no longer dwelled on the physical functionality I was losing, but instead became thankful of what functionality still remained. I began to accept the reality of my incurable chronic heart failure as simply part of the life I was living. With this came a sense of contentment that took hold of my consciousness and changed my attitude toward living. I was now at peace with full acceptance of whatever the future might bring and began to experience a joy that had been missing even before I became ill.

Expectedly my condition continued to deteriorate and subsequently my physician daughter-in-law convinced me to come to Ann Arbor for evaluation. Under the care of the heart doctors at the University of Michigan I did as well as could be expected, but in early 2008 I was hospitalized again, with severe congestive heart failure. Subsequently, a different type of pacemaker (bi-ventricular pacemaker) was inserted to pace both my left and right ventricles to further aid my heart's pumping ability. I was then placed on the heart transplant list shortly thereafter.

Near the end of 2008, I had all but lost my ability to speak because my heart had become so enlarged that it was pressing on a nerve that goes to the vocal chords (voice box). I could only talk in a whisper. I no longer answered the phone or participated in conversations since my voice was almost inaudible. I could still talk in a whisper and considered this a blessing, conscious of individuals that are never able to speak and some never able to hear spoken words their entire lives. These individuals, born with such severe disabilities, never seemed to complain. I could hear, see and talk in a whisper. How could I complain? This was just part of living with my disease. There was no sadness as I had begun to realize happiness and contentment do not depend on extrinsic events and stuff one has, but comes from within, from a change of 'heart' and attitude. Death was no longer to be feared as an end to this journey. I was not due for more from this life than that which I had.

In 2009, my condition had deteriorated further, to the point where I was hospitalized, placed on intravenous drugs to assist my failing heart while waiting for a heart transplant. A heart pump LVAD (left ventricular assist device) had been recommended prior to this hospitalization but the remembrance of Barney Clark's life with a mechanical heart still haunted my thoughts and made me shy away from this option. Over twenty years had passed and there had been many improvements in the technology of implantable mechanical devices to assist failing hearts, but in spite of this I held on to this image of Mr. Clark. My perceived experience of what he went through still affected my feelings and thoughts about mechanical devices in the treatment of heart failure. My physicians assured me of the efficacy of the much newer technology, and a short time later when drugs were no longer working and no heart was available for transplant I agreed to have a mechanical pump surgically placed inside me. This was to be a bridge to buy me more time until a transplant became available. My kidneys were failing now and the only hope for any longevity was to have this procedure performed.

I was taken to surgery and a pump (LVAD) was inserted in my chest and upper abdomen to assist my failing heart. This pump worked well, and unlike my fears related to the memories of Mr. Clark, the quality of my life did improve, rather remarkably. After discharge from the hospital and over the next thirteen months, while remaining on the transplant list, my kidneys returned to normal functioning, my lungs remained free of fluid, I could breathe more easily, and had more energy than I had had in the two preceding years. I was actually walking at a slow pace, distances up to three miles, and my voice had returned as my heart size decreased, relieving the pressure on the nerve to my vocal cord. I could talk again! I was grateful and considered each day a blessing. I remained stable for the next twelve months. Living with the pump had become a new and rewarding experience in my journey with heart failure as the physical quality of my life had improved considerably. The memory of that first mechanical heart and Mr. Clark's 112 days faded along with my fear.

I was actually quite fascinated by this, new for me, technology. I could hear the humming of the pump when I turned my head in a certain direction and I had lost my pulse as the pump moved blood in a continuous, not pulsatile manner as the normal heart does. And with the increased energy and strength I kind of fantasized myself as one of those *Marvel* superheroes or a kind of *Robocop*. I would recharge the batteries to my pump each night, plugging them and myself into an electrical socket to keep the pump working, readying myself for the next day of action.

Going along with me on this new path in life, this journey with heart failure was my co-pilot wife. Her support along with our son, daughter, other family members and friends were acts of pure charity in the Biblical sense. My daughter stayed with me for days after surgery, during which I was severely physically and mentally impaired; my wife was with me every day and many nights; my brother slept on a gurney in the hospital hallway while I was in surgery; my son and his great optimism and my daughter-in-law who had directed me to the doctors at Ann Arbor; and all who kept my family and friends updated about my condition. My son-in-law composed a song about me and my LVAD on an album. And finally the nurses, surgeons and heart doctors, social workers, along with the med techs, nurse-aids, and all the paramedical personal; I cannot say enough about their care. They actually gave me back a better functioning life with my new LVAD friend, "Mr. Pump." Without this heart pump, I would not be here years later as a functional human being. There was much to be thankful for.

Nearing the end of this piece, I must say a few more words about my wife of over 45 years. First of all, I can't imagine what road my life's path would have followed if I had not met and married her, but it certainly would not have been a yellow brick road. She was my guiding light, always steering me in the correct direction with each fork in the road. It was much more difficult and stressful for her as my co-pilot, nurse and caretaker while on this journey. She had to learn the sound of the different alarms from the heart pump indicating certain problems and what to do in each case. She had to learn how to change the dressing where the driveline (a "wire" connected to the pump inside me, through which batteries supplied the power for the pump) came out through the skin on the left side of my abdomen. To do this, she would put on a sterile gown, gloves, and mask, clean the area around the driveline and re-bandage the site. This took time and effort. She was my chauffeur as I was not allowed to drive and she was virtually at my side nonstop for the thirteen months while I was supported and kept alive by "Mr. Pump." When I was very sick in the hospital, she was the one worrying and anxious, much more than me. But this always seems to be the case with a loving spouse. I simply cannot imagine the world without her. I simply would not be the person I am. The LVAD added to and extended that world.

I was now doing well at one year after having my LVAD placed and seeing the doctors only at three-month intervals. I had gained much of my energy and muscle strength back; I was feeling well and fairly functional, though far from how I had been before developing congestive heart failure. After I had turned sixty-five years old and was nearing my sixty-sixth birthday, I felt content to live out what remaining time I had left here on earth with this pump, gratified, satisfied and happy. I thought when I turned sixty-five that my chances of getting a heart transplant were fading. And that was OK by me. I was doing well and others were surely more sick and in need than me.

I was now comfortable and had gained a new appreciation of life that I never ever had before I developed heart failure. This I cannot understate. Before I became ill with heart disease, life was doing things, like skiing, having stuff, amusement, working and having fun. Life was about me.

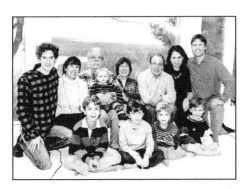

Mike's Family Photo

After the experience of losing my health, my voice and my physical ability, the implanting of my LVAD helped me regain much of this and I came to realize - while we're here on earth, it's relations with family and friends that are really the important things that matter, not stuff, amusements, travel, etc. The joy this has given me with the increased affinity, love and kinship with family and friends seems a gift that I would never have realized had I not become ill with heart disease. Sometimes we have to lose something to gain something.

After thirteen months with my "Mr. Pump," with no infections or complications and actually having gone an entire year without being in the hospital, I often thought of how fortunate I was to be alive and functional. Then at 1:30 am, on December 14th of 2010, I received a phone call indicating that a donor heart had been matched to me. I received a heart transplant later that day.

Joey is my donor's name and I am aware of his heart pumping every hour of every day. I know his life's history from his gracious loving parents. We communicate and meet with them on a regular basis. One can never heal completely from the sudden unexpected loss of one's own child but may have some consolation realizing how much his heart has benefited me, and they seem to sense Joey is with us each time we get together. Joey's mom always takes time to listen to his heart, placing her head on my chest for a short period of time, hearing the sounds of his heart speaking to her while I sense her sorrow and at the same time, my joy and privilege of having received this gift of life. I will honor his heart and memory until the day "we" die and hopefully meet in heaven.

When I first became ill with heart failure, my future was a blur and I had no idea what to expect in terms of longevity. I had read somewhere that having heart failure was similar to having an incurable cancer. Thus, at that time, I had no expectations that I would see my son or daughter marry and have my grandchildren. But years later I was able to walk my daughter down the aisle a few months after transplantation and now have had four grandsons from my son and his wife and two granddaughters from my daughter and her husband. The experience of grandchildren is one like no other; it truly gives meaning to life, experiencing three generations of family with over a 70-year age differential.

This morning, before concluding this narrative of memories, Joey and I took my dog on a 4.4-mile jog in the cool morning. It is during these early morning times that I can pray and thank God for my existence and the consciousness of that existence and beyond. I go early in the morning, often before sunrise when there are few sounds of traffic or other people about. I hear only the sound of my feet hitting the pavement, the jingle of my dog's collar, and feel the beating of a heart I share from another.

I am alive for another day. I am blessed. I give thanks. I have a changed heart.

Verghese

My Heart Story

O ver the past five years, I have been volunteering on various occasions for the Gift of Life organization: speaking to Health Science Seniors at our local high schools (Pioneer & Huron), promoting organ donor registrations at the local Secretary of State office with my daughter and at various venues at the hospitals of the University of Michigan as well as at St. Joes. Prior to that, it would have never occurred to me to be volunteering in this capacity although, I was always pushing my two kids to get into a lifestyle of volunteerism, that is seemingly so prevalent in this great country that we leave in. But life has its ways of throwing you curve balls that over time, even if you have never played baseball, you learn to deal with and surprisingly teach yourself to successfully manage.

Late 2013, I was asked to be the keynote speaker at the annual 2013 Vita Redita Gala Dinner & Auction held at the Michigan Big House. This is the #1 organ donation fundraiser in the State of Michigan. It was going to be a black tie event with many dignitaries, friends of the UM hospitals, surgeons and other hospital staff attending. Once I realized how big this was going to be, I almost tried to back out but it seemed too late for that. In the end I was extremely glad to have been part of this event and to have shared my story. That speech ended in a standing ovation from the crowd and a record amount for donations was gathered that night — a whopping $92,000. But even after doing this now for a while, I am still always a little taken aback when folks ask me to speak for any public occasion. In my mind, I haven't done anything spectacular to warrant any of this. I just happen to be a recent recipient of a donor organ, specifically a new heart, courtesy of the UM Hospital. I didn't win a gold medal, I didn't break any records, I didn't save anyone's life, none of that. In fact, all I did was to get very, very sick over a period of 10 years…so sick, that in Dec 2009 when I came for what I thought was a routine cardiology visit, my cardiologist, Dr. Todd Koelling, told me that my heart had come to its final days and that I wouldn't be going home that night…

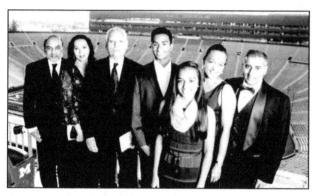

Family photo from the Vita Redita Banquet in 2013 when I was the keynote speaker. From left to right is: Philip (brother-in-law), Leena (sister), T.J. (father), Tristan (son), Nikhita (daughter), Sunita (wife), me

So, let me take you back a little bit from there…I was born in 1963 as the youngest of four siblings in Bombay (now known as Mumbai), India. Due to my father's occupation for the Indian government, we moved a lot. After only three years in India, my entire family left on a ship across the Indian Ocean to Nairobi, Kenya and there we stayed for five years. What a beautiful country, located right on the Equator. From there we moved to Frankfurt, West Germany in 1972 with a six-month stint for me at a boarding school back in India before joining my family again in Germany. So Germany (or West Germany, as it was known while I was there) is basically where my formative youth and teenage years were spent. And this is also where my love for the game of soccer (football as the rest of the world knows it) began.

I bring up soccer because it is very closely tied to nearly everything that has happened to me in life as well as with all my medical issues. Long story short, I was a pretty decent soccer player even though I never really had any formal training in it. I simply honed my skills by playing daily out on the streets, parks, and subway stations in Frankfurt. By the way, my parents never wanted me to play soccer and always discouraged it. Us Indians are all about studies, studies and more studies. When was the last time you saw an Indian with a soccer ball, right?

Well eventually, playing for the Frankfurt International High School in Germany and for a German club during my junior and senior years, I gained some local recognition and my HS coach, who had played in an American college, convinced me to look for a college-level opportunity in the United States. Remember this was the early 80s… no Internet, no video tapes, no YouTube, etc. Thus, my letters from Germany seeking a scholarship opportunity to a US college coach really didn't have any feet to stand on. All I had was a recommendation letter from my HS coach and a list of my various soccer accolades garnered in Europe.

But Fate would see to it that the first ever soccer coach at Eastern Michigan University (EMU) happened to be traveling through Germany and saw me play a game. He encouraged me to come to EMU and walk in to the team and that is exactly what I did. EMU had a Varsity program for soccer and soccer at UM was only a Club sport. So on August 1983, 30 years ago, I left my comfortable life in Germany behind and arrived here in Michigan to start a new adventure. I walked in to the team, earned a scholarship spot and played four years of Div I soccer for the Hurons (yes, not the Eagles)… I was a student-athlete playing my favorite sport and getting a partially free US college education, to boot… LIFE WAS GOOD!

Then life got even better. During my sophomore year I met another foreign athlete at EMU… A tennis star from Barbados, a tiny Caribbean Island. The EMU tennis coach happened to be vacationing in Barbados that summer and happened to see her play in an exhibition and after watching only one set, offered her a full scholarship to come play for EMU. That young girl, Sunita, would eventually become my wife eight years later, with whom I would

… the doctors warned me that when the device would fire, in their own words, 'it would feel like a mule kicking me in the chest.' Since I never had a mule kick me before, I didn't really know what to make of that. But I found out soon enough.

63

have two beautiful children, both of whom are or were also Pioneer HS students.

After Sunita and I completed our Bachelor degrees we went on to receiving Graduate Assistantships at EMU and thus, also completed our Masters degrees there. I received degrees in Computer Science and Business Information Systems. Meanwhile, I kept playing soccer in various local clubs in and around Michigan. Soon we started a family and our son was born in 1995. While I always wanted him to learn the true game on the streets with his friends like I had done so many years ago, I soon realized that it never really could happen that way in the US. While elsewhere in the world, soccer is one of the most inexpensive games to play. Everybody in the world plays the beautiful game in parks, on streets, in alleys, etc. It is truly the common man's sport. However, here in the US, soccer has turned into an extremely organized and relatively expensive sport. While I originally never thought of formally coaching my son, once I saw the alternatives of who actually would be volunteering to coach the Rec-and-Ed teams, I decided I had to step in and coach him. Thus, my stint as a soccer coach began primarily due to guide my son in the correct direction. So from the humble beginnings of a neighborhood boys team that I coached and kept together for seven years, taking them through the club-system with Ann Arbor United, today, five boys from that team have gone on to play at the highest level of youth soccer (USSF Academy Development system) in the US with some of them going on to continue playing in college now.

Well, if I'm here writing about transplants, life can't have been all-good. Something bad must have happened, right? Yes, in November 1999, one week before my daughter, Nikhita, was born, I had my first heart attack. I was only 36 years old! It happened while I was playing soccer. And that was the beginning of all my heart problems. I never even knew that I was having an attack. I just felt some dizziness during the game and it seemed like I was a bit more tired than normal but I simply put it off as being out of shape. So I finished the game and got home very late. Too tired to walk up the stairs, I just laid myself down on the carpet and closed my eyes. Luckily, my wife found me and helped me up to our bedroom. I wasn't feeling any classic chest pains or the elephant sitting on my chest... just a little bit of trouble breathing properly and keeping anything in my stomach. Since it was the flu season, I just thought I was coming down with the flu or something. But since my unborn daughter was expected any day and not wanting to take any risks, it was on a Sunday afternoon that we decided to go to the ER. Remember, my heart attack happened on Friday evening. With hindsight, the doctors now believe that waiting for about 36 hours before getting to the hospital is what eventually worsened my situation and that is when the major damage to my heart tissue occurred.

The EKG verified that I did indeed had an attack on that Friday while playing. Soon word got out amongst some of the other doctors who coincidently also played in some of the same leagues that I played in and knew me well and they went to work on me immediately. Three days before the birth of my daughter, stents were implanted inside two of my arteries, which had about 70% blockages. The strange thing is that while I was having my operation, at the same time in Toronto both my parents were also undergoing heart-bypass surgery. Theirs was scheduled and mine obviously not. So was it a matter of bad genes or merely a freak coincidence? Who knows?

With both my parents recovering, my siblings decided NOT to tell them anything about my condition. Unfortunately, my mother's recovery was not ideal and she passed away two months after the surgery. On the other hand, my father's recovery was one of the best ones they had seen and he was back home after only a little over 1 week. He is still doing great, is very independent, drives on his own and this past June turned 90 years young.

After only a few months of rehab, I was back playing soccer as well as coaching my son's team again. The docs knew that I loved soccer and they never put any restrictions on me. I was free to go about my normal life. Life was good again... but only for a short while.

Four years would pass (2003) by and once again, on the soccer field during a game... I had just dribbled the ball up and made a pass to a teammate... That was the last thing I remembered until I came around to find myself lying on the ground with all my teammates huddled around me. They would later tell me that I was standing one moment and then next I fell over like falling timber, hit my head on the ground and lay motionless. Someone called 911 and I am still amazed at how fast EMS showed up to the field. At first they were asking me a lot of questions and taking my vitals but I kept telling them that I was having difficulty breathing. Lying on the field, they placed a ventilator over my face. This helped initially but I could sense that I wasn't able to get an entire gulp of air into my lungs. A little bit of panic started to set in and I kept telling the first responder that it was getting worse. Boy, I am so glad he knew exactly what he was doing when he sensed that I was fading. He pulled out a syringe filled with some magical potion, yes, to me it was magical, stuck it into my arm and pushed down.

The relief was immediate. I felt this rush of oxygen suddenly surge into my lungs and I could breathe normally again. Up until then, that was the closest I had been to death. Today in my talks that I give, I describe it as the scene from Tarantino's classic, *Pulp Fiction*. I can't tell you how many times I kept thanking the EMS guys while I was being stretchered off the field. Those guys are some of the real Heroes out there amongst us that do this day in and day out.

Once I got to the hospital, Dr. Stan Chetcuti started working on me and implanted another stent to open up a different artery. You know, here in Ann Arbor, it is a small world we live in… Dr. Chetcuti is not only my neighbor but was also the father of one of the boys who I used to coach for

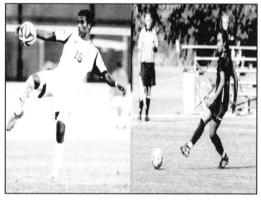

My son (Tristan) and daughter (Nikhita) playing soccer.

several years. Dr. Chetcuti, who is a life-long Liverpool Football Club fan also knew how important soccer was to me, patched me up well.

This time the docs at UM weren't going to take any chances anymore. Several tests and studies were done on me and they eventually figured out what had been going on since my first heart attack. During rigorous exercise as my adrenaline kicked in, my heart would start racing. And when I say racing, I mean a heart rate over 300 beats per minute was not a major feat for me. So, without warming up, from a standstill, if I were to suddenly sprint, my heart rate would approach 300 easily… At those rates, your heart is basically not able to pump any blood to the rest of your body and it is simply quivering. Where in a normal heart when an electrical signal comes in on one side and goes out the other side, which basically signals your heart to create a beat, contract and then pump your blood, in my 'broken' heart, that same electrical signal would come in but then get confused with all my dead tissue inside my heart and then start going round and round in a never-ending loop, thus continuously raising my rate.

I guess the doctors got tired of EMS coming out to rescue me each time I had an incident, so they decided to implant a tiny internal defibrillator, also known as an ICD, right above my heart. While this battery-operated device was supposed to take the place of the EMS, it also changed life for me. From then on, I could never again go through the regular security line at airports, was told not to stay near to security doors, could never get an MRI anymore and particularly, had to always spend about 20 minutes on the treadmill in my basement trying to get my heart warmed up before I could go out and do any sort of high intense sport like soccer. These ICDs operate on a battery whose shelf life was about 5 years then, so I knew that eventually they would have to open me up again to replace it.

When they discharged me, the doctors warned me that when the device would fire, in their own words, 'it would feel like a mule kicking me in the chest.' Since I never had a mule kick me before, I didn't really know what to make of that. But I found out soon enough. During the four years living with the device, there were many, many times when it went off and as with everything else, always during playing or coaching soccer. I had to always wear an athlete's heart strap around my chest and had to get permission from the referees to wear a heart watch whenever I exercised or played soccer, continuously looking at the watch to see if I was approaching the limit. The device was programmed to go off at a heart rate of 190, which is quite high for a normal human, but I had no problems getting it to that level. Each time it fired, I was forced to scream out loud and the sheer force of the electrical jolt would knock me off my feet and I would feel this ringing sound inside my head for about five minutes later. It was just like they showed you in the movies, except that there it was always being done to someone you thought was dead already. In my case, I was fully aware that the shock was coming and even while I knew it, it would knock me down.

Just one year later in 2004, yes, playing soccer again… another incident. This time outdoors at Fuller Park. I was walking over to pick up the ball to throw it in and then it happened again… my teammates told me that when I bent over to pick up the ball, I slowly curled over and hit the ground and lay motionless. They also saw my body shortly thereafter lift off the ground from the force of the ICD shock. Luckily for me, the UM hospital was right across the street and once again EMS came over in no time even though my ICD did its job and revived me. Later when they interrogated my device, they found out that my heart had been beating on the field at the rate of 340 bpm!

Over the years, the ICD had always worked as advertised and applied the all important shock when needed, which would then bring my heart back into a normal rhythm and I would stop whatever I was doing and rest. However, on one occasion in 2007, while playing soccer again, it shocked me once. By now I was fairly used to it and my teammates also knew about these crazy occurrences. So not wanting to cause a scene again, I simply walked off to the bench while everyone else kept playing. Looking at my heart watch, I noticed that my heart rate was still staying fairly high and not coming down. I tried drinking some water but when I realized I was approaching 190 again, I stood up and held on to the bench to brace myself… Sure enough, the second shock came and I had to yell out loud again. First, a few teammates noticed and then quickly everyone stopped the game and came to tend to me, pouring water over me, massaging my neck, etc. One of them had his hand on my shoulder during one of the shocks and he told me later that he also felt the shock go through his body. By now, I had been in and out of Emergency rooms so often that I hated going there. So, while my teammates were about to call 911, I told them to wait a little while longer and that the device would eventually do its job. But I was wrong and it didn't stop. After two more shocks, I finally told them to go ahead and make the 911 call.

EMS came and I was carted off again. Lying on the stretcher in the ambulance on the way to the hospital and in between having my vitals taken and them trying to apply an IV to me, I would have to warn the attendants eight more times to stay away from me as I knew my device well enough to know when it was going to fire. It literally lifted me off the stretcher each time by a few inches. So in total, it went off <u>12 times in those 40 minutes</u>… At the hospital they made adjustments to the device and injected me with some medication to control my heart rate. Shortly thereafter, they performed heart ablation surgery on me to try and burn off the dead areas of my heart tissue in the hope of stopping these extreme loops that the electrical signals would take. That helped for a few months but eventually the crazy rhythms would come back.

As you can imagine, over the years since my first heart attack in 1999, my heart had been taking many beatings (pun intended), for lack of a better word. And like anything else, my heart was slowly wearing down… Ten years after my first heart attack, in December 2009 during a regular checkup visit with my cardiologist, Dr. Koelling had me go through several tests that day. It was a Friday, two weeks before Christmas and I just wanted to get back home even though in the previous weeks and months there were several indications that my kidney and liver functions were degrading and I was in a lot of pain. But you know, it's like when you own a car for a very, very long time… things get old, the engine doesn't run as smoothly as it used to, more noises arise, you take it in for a few tune-ups but in the end, if you can't buy a new car, you just turn up the radio and drown out the noises, right? That was basically what I was doing. When Dr. Koelling came back with the results and told me that my heart was nearing its end, I simply didn't want to believe him. He told me that my Ejection Fraction was so low that he would have to admit me to the hospital. I tried my best to convince him otherwise but eventually my wife also thought it the best path forward.

So I was admitted to the Cardiac Intensive Care unit that night. I assumed they would figure something out to correct the issue and I should be out in a few days. Little did I know that this was going to be my toughest fight I had ever faced. During that night, several more UM cardiologists were consulted and many of them came to analyze my situation. Eventually, they all came together to my room with the bad

I asked my wife to bring our video camera to the hospital and I started making mental notes as to what I wanted to say to my children.

news. Today, this seems so distant now but while I was listening to them, I really didn't comprehend what exactly they were telling me. They basically said that my heart had very little working capacity anymore and the best option they had for me was to perform open-heart surgery and implant a LVAD (Left Ventricular Assist Device) to take over the function of pumping blood to the rest of my body… So here I was, close to death, and all I could think about was that I was NOT going to get back home for Christmas and it sure sounded like they were implying that I wouldn't be playing soccer anymore! It just sounded crazy and even though the docs at UM had taken amazing care of me for all these years, the cynic in me started thinking… you know, these guys see here a guy with good insurance and they are just wanting to try some really expensive procedures on me. Yes, I know now that I wasn't thinking straight then. With all these male doctors surrounding me, it finally took the most soft-spoken female doc (Dr. Audrey Wu) I've ever met, to come in late in the night and speak to me and I finally gave my consent.

On the day before Christmas 2009, Dr. Mathew Romano and his team went to work on me and inserted this mechanical pump inside my body that was to replace my heart function. I'm not sure why but this was the most rigorous and draining procedure I have ever endured in my life. I was in intensive care for over a week. They had tubes coming out of me in every direction. If I thought getting the ICD implanted in me was a major life change, this was going to completely turn my life style upside down. I lost twenty-five pounds within a few weeks of just lying in the hospital bed and every bit of any muscle that I had was nearly all gone. It took me weeks to simply get the strength to get up in bed. Even trying to take a few steps would end up with me collapsing. In total, I spent 41 days in the hospital trying to regain some weight and muscle after forcing myself to eat more protein and slowly walking around the ward with the help of a walking device. I had lost all my taste buds and so eating was very difficult and I would simply avoid it.

Things got so difficult during this time that I already started talking to my wife about plans for the future without me. I asked my wife to bring our video camera to the hospital and I started making mental notes as to what I wanted to say to my children. But there were Heroes around me again… my wife came for daily visits after her work and getting the kids to where they needed to be.

My family from Toronto would also come occasionally to visit me. My daughter wrote me notes and drew pretty pictures for me. My son would come by and chat with me about soccer and how his team was doing. Teammates, neighbors and local friends would continuously stop by, bringing gifts, protein shakes, chitchat and stay for a while.

Once again, it wasn't my time to leave yet and with the support of all these folks, I made it back home. This time around though, the life that I always knew until then had now changed forever. Let me tell you a little about this LVAD unit… I had this good-sized CPU strapped to my waist with blinking lights and different sounds that it made that signaled various different alerts. Connected to this mini-computer was a driveline that went around and into an opening in my stomach and continued on to the actual LVAD pump inside of me. Of course, the brains of this device had to get its juice from somewhere right? Let me tell you, we are not talking about some triple-A batteries either. It was always connected to these two things that looked like bricks and weighed as much as well, which would hang down from my side in these holsters that were also on the strap. Every few hours the batteries would have to be changed with new ones, while the old ones charged up in a stand-by unit and thus all this equipment had to be with me at all times. While sleeping at night, I removed the batteries and then plugged myself into the wall outlet. Each night, my wife had to put on a surgical mask, suit and gloves to minimize chances of infecting me, and then disinfect the opening of at my stomach where the driveline went in, and then bandage everything up again. I was not allowed to bring any water around the opening for fear of infections. That meant no showers! I can tell you that using washcloths daily is not easy and no fun. All this went on every day for six months.

Part of the agreement to get an LVAD is that you also have to have someone with you at all times. Well, that can be quite tricky if you don't have a large family around you. So while my wife was at work during the day, my sister, Leena, put her job in Toronto on hold and stayed with us for the first few weeks. I then set up a walkie-talkie system going on with one of my neighbor, Anna Dutton, just in case any of the alarms went off. I also was not allowed to drive anymore and since this was now in the winter I would get driven to Briarwood Mall or to the local Meijer and I would slowly walk around trying to gain more strength. Additionally, since there were some complications during the surgery with some blood flow to me feet, I was condemned to wearing a large foam boot on one foot and use a walking cane to get around. This was a far cry from the active father and soccer player I had been all my life. After about three months, I started working part-time from home again and slowly tried driving again even though I wasn't really supposed to. I've always been an independent person and I just couldn't be locked up like this at home. Slowly but surely, I got strong enough where I became eligible to get on the transplant waiting list.

By now, I had come to accept that this was my fate and that I had to make the best of it. But believe it or not, that was OK with me. You know at least I was alive and still with my family and I was extremely grateful for that. But one of the things I missed most was watching my kids play soccer. Thus, I got several friends and team parents trained and certified on the various LVAD alerts, which then allowed me to drive with them to my children's soccer games.

Then in late June 2010, only six months after the LVAD was implanted, my son, who by then was starting to become a very good player in his own right, club soccer team (Michigan Wolves) had just won the State Championship and were moving on to the Midwest Regional Finals… Well, I wasn't about to miss seeing that so I messed up. I had forgotten that I was told not to travel more than two hours away from UM, now that I was on the transplant list for a new heart. So, contrary to the doctor's advice, I got both my kids trained on the LVAD functions and all three of us drove to Dayton, Ohio to watch my son play.

We came back to the hotel after his first game and I was watching TV with my daughter when I received a phone call. It was actually **THE** phone call. I was surprised because the call was from a friend and mother of a former player of mine who I had coached for several years (small world again). Ms. Kathy Bartos was a transplant coordinator working with the UM Transplant Unit at the time and she wanted to personally give me the good news. Now understand, that by this time now, I had gotten used to dealing with my LVAD and just thinking about the ordeal I went through for that operation, really didn't make the thought of another operation seem very desirable. I actually told Kathy that I didn't really want to do this now. I told her that I was OK living my life with these restrictions. She got very serious on the phone and said that there were hundreds of people waiting for years to get a young heart like this and I should NOT pass up this chance. She told me that the docs had specifically waited for a very young heart because of how active I was. Well, I finally agreed but I had to tell her that I was in Ohio, more than three hours away from Ann Arbor. But Kathy was adamant. She just told me to not to worry, to get in the car and drive as fast as I could back to the UM hospital. She said they would do everything to keep the heart alive for me.

So I left my son behind with some of the other parents and took my daughter with me for the drive back to keep me company. Remember I told you that I grew up in Germany? Well, I also got my training for my driver's license on the German Autobahns. I think I made the trip back to Ann Arbor in little more than 2.5 hours. Someone must have been looking out for me because not a single Ohio trooper stopped me. I was hoping to talk to my daughter during the ride but ten minutes into it and she was fast asleep. So while driving I called my wife, my family in Toronto and some close friends to tell them all what was going on because I was really nervous.

We came back home, took just the bare necessities, dropped Nikhita off at our neighbor's home and made it to the CVC in record time. My wife and I were then briefed on the procedure and I was carted away. My old hero, Dr. Mathew Romana who had implanted the LVAD in me was there again and I believe the entire operation took only 5 hours and went into the night. Apparently, I slept for an entire day after the operation and woke up to bright sunshine in another room. This time it was nothing like after the LVAD surgery. The nurse helped me up from the bed and I could walk on my own immediately. I took a peek under my gown at my chest and it was all bandaged up but my LVAD, the driveline and the batteries were all gone. Unbelievable I thought!!!!

They took my broken heart out, got rid of all the implanted stents, the LVAD and replaced everything with this young pristine heart from a complete stranger. And obviously, you can't just take one heart and put another one in at the exact same time, right. So, for some period of time, I was lying there without a heart and being sustained by a machine. I am still amazed as to everything these docs can do.

Prior to this, the docs and nurses had always told me that heart transplants were very routine at UM and there was very little to worry about. Sure enough, I stayed in the hospital for only twelve days and then was released to leave. Being off now from work again and with the nice summer weather, I started to walk every day in our cul-de-sac, round and round in circles.

A few weeks later, I started riding my bike around the neighborhood, then slowly jogging and then finally running and sprinting again. Being able to sprint again was just so amazing to me. So I got the new heart on June 27th. Exactly two months later, I was back on the soccer field again… and I was running and playing like I hadn't done in over seven years. I was always worried that something would happen to this new heart if I play really hard so I would take it easy in the beginning. But it just kept on beating and it never went into those crazy rhythms and slowly I started pushing myself harder and harder. I then realized that the only thing holding me back were my 50-year old knees.

Think about it, a tragedy occurred somewhere on June 27th. Some family lost a son, someone may have lost a brother, a cousin or a nephew. The survivors were deep in grief and sorrow over their loss, arguably the worst moment of their lives. But exactly during that time they found it in their hearts to fulfill their dead son's last wish to donate his organs. I was told that on that same night, both his lungs were used for someone else in need at UM also.

The Power of Organ Donation.

In the midst of such a tragedy, I got another chance at life, to see my son and daughter grow up and a chance for my wife to have her husband again. I was

In the midst of such a tragedy, I got another chance at life, to see my son and daughter grow up and a chance for my wife to have her husband again.

able to see my son go on to play for the Major League Soccer (MLS) team, Columbus Crew's Academy and also my daughter make the Michigan Olympic Development Program (ODP) team as one of the twenty-two best players in the state for her age group. She has also gone on to make the USA National Futsal U16-U18 team, representing them in Costa Rica this past summer and currently playing at the highest level of club soccer for girls in the US.

Remember, I also mentioned that several kids that I had coached over the years had gone on to play at the collegiate level? Well, in 2012, the University of Michigan Wolverine Varsity Soccer team, under then a 2nd-year head coach, Chaka Daley, saw enough of my son's playing ability and ended up recruiting him for the incoming class of 2014. Today, Tristan is a proud member of the Wolverines team and has never regretted his choice.

You know the world today is very different from when my wife and I came to play here in the US… no one interviewed us, followed us on Twitter or had highlight videos of us on YouTube, etc. But it was very different for my son during his recruiting days. I found out about this only later but after he verbally committed to Michigan in 2012, he was interviewed by an Internet online magazine and one of the questions they asked him was why he finally chose Michigan over the other schools which were also interested. What he said left me speechless for a while… To paraphrase Tristan: Besides, being a great school and him feeling very comfortable with Coach Daley and some of the guys already on the team, he said that he really wanted to do something to pay back UM for saving his father's life.

So in the end, I would like to thank Ms. Ruth Halben for allowing me to share my story with all of you. I can't say enough Thank-Yous to the many doctors that took care of me and still do today and to all those unsung heroes like the members of the EMS crews.

I specifically want to give a BIG HUG to all those hard working nurses, who never let me sleep an entire night without waking me up to get my vitals, but without whom I would not have made it.

But if there's one thing I would like you to take away from my story, it is to know that there is no major religion on the planet that asks you to take your physical body with you when you leave this world. Each of us has nine organs that we could donate to save potentially nine other lives. All you need when you get up there is your spirit and your soul. Leave your vital organs here for those who need them most. We all know how many people fit the Big House. Now think about the list of people on the waiting list for an organ transplant. That list is larger than any record-breaking crowd ever to fit in that stadium.

Please consider going to the Secretary of State in the near future and put your names on the Donor List and get your red heart sticker on your driver's license.

THANK YOU.

Bill

A Birthday Wish

In November of 2000, I found myself unable to sleep through the night. This had been going on for several months and finally my wife convinced me to see my internist. I made an appointment and saw my friend Dr. Robert Ernst the next week. Initially, I wasn't very concerned because my health was generally pretty good. At that time, I had a great job and I felt like I had the world by the tail.

Dr. Ernst came in and as usual he asked me what was going on. I described my lack of sleep and ongoing feeling of fatigue. We talked about the extensive travel required by my job and whether there was any way to cut back. I emphatically refused because cutting back would mean that I had to give up some of the responsibility that made me king of the world. He said he wanted to run some tests and I'd be there for a while.

When he said he wanted to run some tests he wasn't kidding. I spent three hours in his office that morning. When I finally came back in I could see the look on his face. He asked me questions about anyone in my family having a history of heart disease. I told him no. He said that while he was not a cardiologist, he was pretty sure that his diagnosis would prove to be correct. He told me that, from all the test results, it appeared that I had an enlargement of the heart indicative of cardiomyopathy. I consider myself a very bright guy, but I had no idea what that meant. He explained that my left ventricle was failing and was having a difficult time supplying the proper blood flow to my organs. I MUST HAVE LOOKED LIKE I HAD BEEN SLAPPED WITH A BASEBALL BAT BECAUSE clearly he could see the astonishment on my face. So now the real questions began. He told me that he wanted me to begin to take four different medications immediately and to see a cardiologist within the next two days. I naively asked him what I should have left alone – how long I would be taking medication. He looked at me and said that I would be on medication for the rest of my life. For a guy like me that felt like a death sentence.

On the drive home I tried to figure out how I was going to share this with my wife. We had been married for over twenty years and had just sent our only child off to college. I arrived home, and before I could get my coat off, she wanted to know what Dr. Ernst had said. I sat her down and told her and then made the appointment with the cardiologist. Needless to say there wasn't a lot of talking going on at home that day. I was already beginning to anticipate the worst.

A couple of days later, I had my consultation with the cardiologist. He did not have a very positive bedside manner. He reviewed Dr. Ernst's findings and concurred with his diagnosis. He then told me that it was his opinion that I had about twenty-four months to live. He referred me to the Heart Failure and Transplant unit at the University of Michigan. That was the best thing he could have done for me.

In January of 2001, I started seeing Dr. John Nicklas. In our first visit, I told him what the other cardiologist had said about my prognosis and he told me to forget about it. He said I was clearly much sicker than I thought I was, but that in and of itself was not a death sentence. We repeated a lot of the tests from earlier and found that my ejection fraction was less than fifteen. We talked about what I did for a living and how that was likely to impact my health.

On the drive home I tried to figure out how I was going to share this with my wife. We had been married for over twenty years and had just sent our only child off to college.

From that point on, Dr. Nicklas became my cardiologist. I began to see him once or twice a month to monitor how I was doing. In March of 2001, I took a long-term medical leave of absence because I just couldn't do it anymore. Dr. Nicklas was in total agreement. I thought I just needed a rest and he thought that trying to go back would be the kiss of death.

He turned out to be right. In July, I went back to work and within a month, I was downsized after years of being a superstar. That was hard for my ego to take. With medication, my condition stabilized and until 2006 things went pretty much according to plan. In the fall of 2006, I had my first of two ICD implanted. You can't keep a good guy down.

In 2008, I took a job as the CEO of SurfRay, a Danish software company. On one of my trips to Denmark I received an emergency call that my defibrillator was acting erratically. I jumped on a plane and flew back that evening. The next day I received a replacement device because the wires had worked themselves loose. Kind of scary! By the end of 2008, I found a larger software company to purchase SurfRay and once again was unemployed. 2009 was like running downhill at full speed. My health had started a precipitous decline. My renal function was adversely impacted and increasing my diuretic was not an option.

In January of 2010, I started having a Vo2 study every six weeks and every six weeks the study showed a decline. Dr. Nicklas, who I now considered not just my doctor but a friend, was honest in telling me that I had reached the end of what pharmaceuticals could do to control the problem. I was scheduled for a clinic visit on June 10th when Mary, Dr. Nicklas' nurse, called and told me to bring my bag because I probably would not be going home. I got to the clinic and Dr. Nicklas told me he needed to admit me that day. Even though I had brought my bag I was not prepared to hear that. Being the type A that I am, I tried to bargain about coming back the next Monday. He wasn't having it. He broke out the big guns. He told me that I was functioning on borrowed time, and that unless we did something immediately, I probably wouldn't last six months.

I was admitted to the hospital and thus began the LVAD discussion. I should be perfectly honest and say that it was a non-starter for me. I wasn't interested.

Everybody over the next week came in to see me – Dr. Nicklas, Dr. Wu, Dr. Koelling, everybody! Finally, they brought in God, Dr. Pagani. He proceeded in his non-passionate way to read me the riot act. I spent a week saying no. After a lot of heartfelt thought and consideration, I relented. On the morning of June 21st, 2010, I was implanted with the Heartmate II LVAD device.

My initial reaction was not positive. I didn't like the restrictions it made on my life. But it kept me alive. I got to meet a very special friend, John Flynn, who was implanted after I was. John's courage and fortitude put me to shame. John didn't make it, but in the short time we had to know each other, I learned to love and respect him. I miss him every day.

When I got my LVAD my own father was 98 years old. He was more worried about me than about himself. Throughout this journey I have learned so many things. The week of my father's 99th birthday we had planned a birthday party for him. That week I had felt pretty crummy and on several occasions we had considered canceling the party. We went ahead with it and I think he really enjoyed himself.

By the time our last guest left, I was bone weary. I immediately climbed into bed. At 2:00 AM that morning, the phone rang. None of us ever look forward to those calls. It was the transplant unit at U of M calling to say they had a heart for me. To say that I was speechless would be an understatement.

I picked up the phone and called my father. He didn't say anything for what seemed like forever. When he finally spoke he said that he had received his birthday wish. My wife and I got my things together and drove up to U of M. When they wheeled me into the operating room I can honestly tell you that I have never felt such a sense of peace. I was not afraid.

I was transplanted on May 8th, 2011. It continues to be a journey, and I wouldn't trade it for anything in the world. I've lived to see my son graduate from college and earn his master's degree. I've met my donor's family and now I have a new extended family. No one knows the toll that this work takes on you people who dedicate your lives to saving others. God bless you and keep you. You are truly his angels!

Clayton

With Heartfelt Thanks

Hi, my name is Clayton, (Clay) age 65. My road to recovery started late 1998 when I was told that I had A-fib and that my left ventricle was deteriorating. At the time a heart transplant seemed to be out of question. So I got on with my life. We moved to northern Michigan and built our retirement home. The next few years were spent building our new life. I was ignoring the fact that I was getting shorter of breath and tiring much faster. All the while thinking I would finish this and it would be there for my wife and family. Boy, how things change!

My cardiologist in Traverse City recommended that I see the heart group at the University of Michigan. We knew their reputation and had no qualms about going there. The cardio team at U of M followed my heath for a couple years, and it was progressively getting worse. By that time, my heart and I were ready to meet the rest of the cardio team. They decided to put a left ventricle assist device (LVAD) in my heart to help it pump the blood out and to keep me on an even keel as long as possible. I learned that at that time, there was no other option for me and so the journey began.

My LVAD experience started with me and my family being concerned, but glad we were moving along toward a solution to my health problems. We were told that in my case having the LVAD was the next step before having a heart transplant.

My LVAD operation was one of life's little bumps, the recovery was the hard part. It took a while for many reasons, one being a fall. In the middle of the night I needed to use the restroom. Well, me being the impatient person I am, I got out of the bed, started for the bathroom, (bad move) I landed on the floor, IV and all, biting my tongue very badly and darn near ruined all the work the nice Docs had done. The wonderful nurses rescued me and put me back in bed and told me to stay there, unless accompanied by one of them.

During the operation, I had two mini strokes and wasn't able to swallow food, so I had to have a tube down my throat to get fed. Unfortunately, I had to go home with the tube, but everything else concerning my health was fine.

This part was a little scary for me and for my wife, as she was told that she was going to have to feed me with the tube. Luckily, my daughter was involved with every aspect of the education on the operation and the training that U of M provided for my caregivers and myself. That gave my wife a chance to get back to work part-time and get a little time away from it all for a while. Not bad for two people with no background in the medical field.

I won't go into detail about every aspect of the recovery, especially the mental aspect of it but here's to say, it wasn't the best time of my life. But I made it through and one year later, I *got the call we had been waiting for!*

A new heart, wow! We were "afraid" and grateful. My wife and daughter loaded me and my LVAD equipment in the car and we were on our way to U of M. The thoughts running in my head on the drive there were mixed with anxiety and anticipation. Afraid of maybe leaving my wife and family forever, what would happen to "me" with someone else's heart, would it work, would I survive? Even though the professionals at U of M explained everything to me about the procedure. Soooo many doubts and unknowns were running through my head. The trip was many miles (270) long and was covered in such a short time, as the speed limit meant nothing to Mary or my daughter, who pushed Mary faster.

Then came the time for my family to wait and worry. Heck, there was no need for concern. Dr. Romano and his team are very good and have performed this operation many times. My family spent the time praying, going to cafeteria, touring the hospital and watching the flight that brought my heart to me. My daughter in-law knows the people from Med Flight, as she is a flight nurse herself. While I, on the other hand, was out like a faulty light! After hours of nervous waiting, Dr. Romano came out and told my family that everything went very well and that they would see me soon.

The surgery and recuperation from the heart transplant went extremely smooth and I thank the GREAT doctors and nurses at U of M for all the excellent care and the knowledge they have. I also would like to acknowledge the special people "behind the main event" that made my hospital stay and recuperation as easy as possible. Foremost, the people of 4c. I love you all!

I have been a donor all my life and still find it hard to accept the fact that I am now a recipient. How great it is to know that there are people willing to help others. Thank you to all who make the decision to donate their or a loved one's organs. The decision is a difficult one, but the result makes life possible for so many people in need.

We now live in North Carolina and we went to several hospitals and finely found Wake Forest. Wake Forest is a close second to the U *(I compare all to U of M)*. Leaving U of M was a difficult decision, but one I had to make. So here we are in North Carolina, happy & healthy.

I now do almost everything I did before the operations but much easier, which is great because I know my second life is going to be a good one! I feel what was given to me, was nothing short of a miracle and I will do what it takes to make my life as long and happy as possible!

Would I do it again… sure…in a HEARTbeat!

> **I have been a donor all my life and still find it hard to accept the fact that I am now a recipient. How great it is to know that there are people willing to help others. Thank you to all who make the decision to donate their or a loved one's organs.**

I now volunteer at Wake Forest Hospital on Monday and Wednesday and I see all types of heart patients, mostly VAD and Transplants. It's been over a year now and for me it's been very rewarding. I have made some good friends & I have been a part of many transitions' from VAD to transplant. The great part is seeing the patients and their spouses go through the process, their hopes and journey. I can do this because of all the good people of University of Michigan.

My hope is my donor is watching.

Jerome

Looking Healthy

I have been a heart patient for about twenty-three years. My primary care physician first diagnosed me with cardiomyopathy when I did not have enough energy to follow my daily routine. I thought that maybe I was out of shape and needed to exercise to improve my strength and stamina, so I went to see my primary care physician before starting to work out. This was on a Thursday.

He had me take a stress test on a treadmill. I did not make it past phase two, so I was scheduled for some tests in the hospital the following Monday. Over that weekend, I had stomach pains and called my physician's office. I was told to go to the ER at one of our local hospitals. I found out that I was carrying excess water and had cardiomyopathy. For the next fifteen years, my physician and cardiologist treated me with medicine, until I started getting weaker again. That was when I was referred to the U of M hospital. I met with Dr. Todd Koelling. He and my primary care physician co-managed my care with medications and a defibrillator to manage my heart failure.

I became stable and was back to my regular routine. For a while, I felt stronger; but as time went on, I started to feel weaker. That's when Dr. Koelling felt that an LVAD would help give me my strength back. The LVAD would be a bridge to a heart transplant.

On May 2, 2013, Dr. Francis Pagani put in my LVAD. I was in the hospital for thirteen days after the procedure. Before I could leave the hospital, my wife and I had to be able to take my controller apart and put it back together. We had to understand each alarm and what to do if an alarm went off. We learned how to read the battery life screen and how to tell if the batteries were fully charged. I feel like the luckiest man in the world. All of my doctors have been good to me, from my primary care physician all the way through the surgical team. Their communication has been great and they really care. The LVAD people have been wonderful too — it's almost like having another family. I talk to them often and they are always available when I need them. When I do call, the nurses answer all of my questions.

My recovery was pretty quick because I'm in really good shape. I've been with my physical trainer since I was diagnosed twenty-two years ago. When I was first released from the hospital, my trainer spoke to the LVAD people in the clinic. My weakness was apparent at first, but soon my trainer told me I was getting stronger and I had more stamina. I'm not only doing physical training, but also playing golf in a league every week. I also go through antique malls and shows. My wife lets me be as active as I want to be as long as I'm not over-doing it.

I've been able to put a lot of people at ease because, even though they notice the pump in my chest, they can see that I'm back to normal. I get around well and my color has come back. I look and feel much healthier. It's amazing how healthy you can look when blood is flowing through your body the way it should. I feel blessed that I am still here. If I hadn't had the LVAD put in when I did, there's a chance I wouldn't be here today.

> **I've been able to put a lot of people at ease because, even though they notice the pump in my chest, they can see that I'm back to normal... It's amazing how healthy you can look when blood is flowing through your body the way it should.**

86

Ken

LVAD

Hi. I have been putting this off for about six weeks now, probably due to laziness, but I don't really know why. Since my entering the LVAD program I seem to be quite the procrastinator. I am now exhibiting some signs of slight internal bleeding so I would like to get this done before I might have to go to the hospital again. I'm not sure I am doing this in a way that would be advantageous to anyone, but perhaps I will learn something. When I was younger I could write fairly well, but it WILL be interesting to see how this turns out.

My name is Ken. (I am imagining a group of people waving and saying, "Hi Ken".) I am a white male, 70 years old. In my early childhood I grew up in Brooklyn, New York. Growing up there in the 1940s and 1950s was wonderful. We were very poor but everyone else in our neighborhood was also. I had no idea that my life was anything exceptional. But someone once wrote a book about

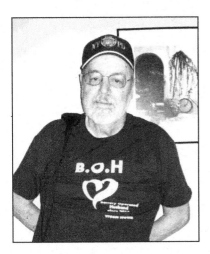

Ken up North;
BOH = battery operated husband

87

growing up there and it was called "We Had Everything But Money." How true. Anyway, as I grew up I always made friends with smokers and drinkers. That became my lifestyle for many decades and it put me where I am today. Tethered with a LVAD, with lung, kidney, and liver damage. It is that reason why I am not eligible for a transplant.

I never said, "Why me?" because I know the answer to that. There have been guilty feelings because I thought I was fairly healthy when I got married in 2000. I have had an absolutely wonderful life and my wife is what I always say, the icing on the cake. I have traveled quite a bit and we were both looking forward to many trips. We did make a few before I got sick but the grand trips I had in my head are now almost impossible.

(This is more intense than I thought it would be. I was expecting to sit here and knock it off in an hour or so. This is how far I got in about an hour and I stopped to take a break. It is now the next day.)

I think that just about anyone reading this is aware of the physical downsides to this situation, but I will briefly mention them just to keep my mind on track for now. I am constantly connected to electricity, either by tether or by batteries. When I go anywhere I have to tote a backup set of batteries and a backup controller. These are not D cells. I must be taped up when I want to take a shower because I cannot afford to let my bandage get wet. There are bacteria even in 'pure' water and an infection would possibly be fatal. Or at least another trip to the hospital for a cleansing and possible another operation. I cannot go swimming and I don't want to chance boating.

For me this is difficult because my greatest joy is spending time at the beach or boating. I am tired a lot and I cannot accomplish things like cleaning the garage or having a garden. It has been said that I should be able to do these things, but it is really very difficult. Before the pump, I would spend eight hours or so cleaning the garage or doing the lawn and flowers. Now, when I spend an hour being active, I become very tired, and usually only accomplish about 15 minutes' worth of activity of pre-pump work. I used to do a lot of painting but I can hardly lift my hands over my head for more than a minute. When I go shopping

I use the cart as a walker and stop frequently to rest my legs. This is not always the case. Usually after some bleeding and my hemoglobin is low.

We lived in the Traverse City area and we really loved it. Plenty of water and wildlife. A photographer's dream. My cardiologist told me that I was getting worse and I would need the pump. We moved to southern Michigan and I checked into the hospital in October 2013.

I already had bleeding problems, lung damage, kidney damage, and liver damage. It took a month for one of the doctors to decide to do the operation. I thank him in my mind with God almost daily, as I do my wife. She is the most wonderful thing that has happened to me and I have had a wonderful life. She is the icing on a seven-layer cake. I digress. After the operation my bleeding problems continued for several months. I was discharged on Christmas Eve and had to return and be re-admitted the next day. Same thing happened on New Year's Eve. Except I stayed home for 3 days before I had to go back. It took a few more weeks and many tests before they did find the source of the bleeding and corrected it. I was very despondent because I did not want to leave my wife alone. We had just moved and the finances were not as good as they are now. I still worry about her finances if I leave. My pension will be lost and she will take my social security but lose hers.

I was home for a year without bleeding of consequence and January of 2015 I had to return to the hospital. I was expecting to go back for treatment every few months but I was lucky. A year off and I forgot about the bleeding. Just kept taking my meds and doing some exercise. My bleeding was corrected in January. I was sent home and in March there was more bleeding. Back for a week and once again I was sent home.

That brings me up to today. Mentally, I have become quite listless. I seem to be content with spending my time on line. I start many projects, but finish very few. I

Mentally, I have become quite listless. I seem to be content with spending my time on line. I start many projects, but finish very few. I am not unhappy, but my wife feels that I am depressed. I don't think so.

am not unhappy, but my wife feels that I am depressed. I don't think so. I thank God just about every day for being alive and I thank Linda every day for tolerating being my caregiver. I thank U of M for their excellent medical care. I seem to be obsessed with death but not necessarily mine. There were periods in the past two years where I became very irritable. Perhaps it was some meds, perhaps it was my circumstances, or perhaps it is frequent in people in my health situation. I don't know, but I do know that I am working very hard to become the person I was before now. I am a bit more pleasant now and I feel good for that.

Well I hope I covered everything of any importance. I hope this is legible. I hope that someone can glean something from this. I have tried to be honest. I think the tone of this statement is more or less negative, but I am adjusting and I am definitely glad for the added time that I have here with my wonderful family. As time goes on I am slowly selling some possessions that I know my wife wouldn't know what to do with after I am gone. And I am going through thousands of pictures and sending negatives and prints of people from my past.

They are no good to my wife and this way she won't have to worry what to do with them.

In any event, I am not sad about the way things turned out up to now. I feel bad because I don't want to see my wife alone. I am slowly getting things in order.

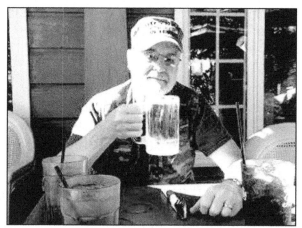

Ken's last drink before LVAD

Dakota

LVAD is Serious

I t all started about one year after I was released from the Toledo Hospital. I was there for treatment after a serious car accident on August 25, 2011. I had episodes that included stomach pain, nausea, dry heaving and heat flashes. Constantly, I was taken to U of M so they could try and figure out what was going on. They eventually diagnosed me with cardiomyopathy, which makes it hard for the heart to deliver blood to the body and can lead to heart failure.

The doctors thought that it would be best to have a pacemaker/defibrillator inserted. After that, I started to feel more like myself again. But that only lasted a short while and unfortunately the original symptoms started arising again. My doctors really didn't want to do any serious treatment, like surgery, right away but it eventually came to that point. Now I have an LVAD, a left ventricular assist device, which is used for patients who have reached end-stage heart failure. I had surgery for the LVAD in February 2015. It has made me feel so much better! I am able to do things I used to do, such as golfing, going on walks, shooting basketball and just hanging out with my friends without feeling sick the whole time. I felt so good that I started slacking on taking my medications and not going to my weekly blood draws. I hadn't felt that good in so long that I somewhat forgot that my condition was so serious.

On July 18th, during my 22nd birthday, my LVAD set off an alarm for HIGH WATTS. I tried telling myself that it was nothing and that I would be fine…but it continued to alarm. The next day, I decided to call the LVAD Emergency phone number and they told me to come right to U of M, as it was possible I had a blood clot in my pump…and they were right.

Shortly after being admitted to the CVC, they tried feeding me 'blood clot fighters' to destroy the blood clots but, unfortunately, it didn't work. My surgeon informed that I did indeed have a blood clot in my pump BUT I also had blood clots in my heart. I would need a very serious surgery. There was no promise that I would make it through the surgery or that I wouldn't suffer from a stroke afterwards. I was scared out of my mind, I couldn't believe that I let this happen. I couldn't believe that my surgeon told me that he would 'try' to get me through this. I just couldn't believe anything that was going on.

Thankfully, I got through the surgery, but this recovery didn't go as smoothly. I suffered both acute kidney failure and acute liver failure. My body was also holding so much water that it got to the point that I was only allowed one liter of fluid a day because the doctors were afraid the excess water would cause me to have seizures. I remained in the hospital for more than 50 days.

This hospital stay was a turning point for me. I realized this condition was serious and that I needed to take control of my life and get my priorities straight. After FINALLY getting home, I made sure I took all of my medications daily, kept up on getting them filled at the pharmacy and went to get my blood drawn weekly.

Anything I was unsure about, I made sure to call the LVAD team to ask about it. Because I started making good and more responsible decisions, I am awaiting approval to be on the heart transplant list. I have started the process by taking my medications to prepare my body for a new heart. Finally, it's happening for me and I can't thank the heart team at U of M enough for everything they have done for me.

Frequently Asked Questions
By LVAD Patients

1) **Can you go swimming with a VAD?**

   Currently none of the VAD's we implant at the University of Michigan will allow you to submerge under water.

2) **Can you shower with a VAD?**

   You are able to shower when you get permission from your surgeon. You will have to protect the external VAD equipment and driveline site as directed by your VAD coordinator.

3) **Can I be sexually active with a VAD?**

   Yes, you may resume sexual activity once you have recovered from your surgery.

4) **Can I drive a car with a VAD?**

   Your surgeon or cardiologist will discuss this with you at your three-month return visit. They will be looking at your post op recovery and any alarm or equipment issues. They may set limitations on where you can drive.

5) **Can I ever be alone (without a caregiver)?**

   Our surgeons and cardiologist prefer you have strong caregiver support, especially in the early post-operative period (first three months). This will be reassessed three to six month after your implant, looking at how well you have recovered and can respond to emergency situations (trouble shooting alarms).

6) How long do we have to do the driveline dressing change?

The driveline always requires a sterile dressing over the site. You or your caregiver will start out having to change it daily for approximately three months then you should be transitioned to a weekly change, as long as there are no issues with the site.

7) Do I have to carry all this VAD equipment with me everywhere I go?

Because your VAD is a life sustaining device it is imperative that you always have your back up controller and fully charged batteries with you at all times.

8) Who will help me troubleshoot VAD equipment issues?

Your VAD team has someone on call 24 7 to assist with medical as well as equipment emergencies. Make sure you and your caregivers always have the on-call number available.

9) Will my local EMS and Fire Department know anything about my VAD?

Your VAD team notifies your local emergency room and first responders when you are discharged home from the hospital. The VAD team answers questions and provides education material; however, it is always a good idea to visit them yourself. Seeing a real patient and equipment is always helpful.

10) How long do these heart pumps last?

That is a complicated question with a lot of different variables that your surgeon will go over with you before your implant. These devices are meant to either bridge you to a heart transplant (if you are a candidate) or extend your life and improve your heart failure symptoms. There are patients out over ten years with VAD's.

Psychosocial Factors of Left Ventricular Assist Device (LVAD) Candidate Selection and Success

"Patient selection for left ventricular assist device (LVAD) therapy is the most important process in obtaining a successful outcome ... additional areas of focus and assessment that can impact adversely on LVAD outcomes include the degree of family and psychosocial support and preoperative neurologic function."

- Aaronson, M.D., Patel, M.D., Pagani, M.D., 2002

Social Support

Candidates for LVAD implantation at University of Michigan are required to have a plan for twenty-four-hour supervision by trained caregiver(s). The caregiving plan must be sustainable for a minimum of 3 months post hospital discharge. There is the potential for 24-hour supervision indefinitely if there are post-operative complications. This plan may consist of a single caregiver or a combination of more than one person, but all must be stable adults, eighteen and older.

The quality of the support system relationships (i.e. primary caregiver, immediate family members, extended family, friends and community) are assessed by the clinical social worker. The patient and identified caregivers' level of stress and coping (strengths or weakness) are considered. Personality characteristics and sense of maturity are also important.

One aspect of support provided by the caregiver(s) is transportation, as the implanted patient is restricted from driving for a minimum of three months. Other aspects of practical support include attendance at clinic appointments or testing, daily or weekly driveline dressing changes, and assistance with medication organization and with equipment.

Emotional support is another necessary part of caring for someone with an LVAD. Both the patient and the caregiver(s) are making a major adjustment to lifestyle and role changes. Coping with these changes can bring about anxious or depressed responses in either the caregiver or the patient.

Other Psychosocial Indicators

Financial

Patients need to have the financial means to be successful with an LVAD, including adequate insurance. Both Medicare and Medicaid cover LVAD surgery. Supplies and medications for the long-term management of the LVAD are often covered, though copays vary depending on insurance coverage.

Some patients receive disability benefits either from an employer paid policy or by qualifying for Social Security Disability. Some patients are able to return to their former employment and some are not, depending on the type of work they were engaged in.

Mental Health

Stable mental health is very important for both the patient and their caregiver(s). Treatment history, willingness to engage in treatment currently, and recent or history of suicidal ideation are considered as they can impact patient compliance

Coping Style

Dealing with major illness and treatment is difficult. Consequently, it is important to develop positive coping strategies. Concerning patterns that impact medical care will be addressed, but would not necessarily be considered a contraindication to LVAD candidacy.

Violence

Domestic violence or other legal issues are considered as they could interfere with one's ability to comply with medical treatment.

Substance Abuse

Smoking and alcohol are not absolute contraindications in destination LVAD implantation, however, if the patient is being considered for heart transplantation, these substances are strictly prohibited and six months of abstinence is monitored with random urine screening. The use of illegal drugs is an absolute contraindication for both LVAD implantation and heart transplantation. Of note, certain over the counter medications may be contraindicated as well. One's history of treatment for substance use and abuse is assessed. The impact of substance abuse could be life threatening.

Cognitive Function
Patients presenting with neurocognitive deficits will be referred for neurocognitive testing and recommendations for patient teaching.

Health Literacy and Compliance
Patients and their caregivers must have the ability to correctly identify and manage medications, as well as VAD equipment and alarms. They must also possess the ability to manage multiple appointments and follow medical and social work recommendations. Knowledge of a healthy diet is also important. Patients and their caregivers are required to review our Success Contract, which specifically outlines the practical side of LVAD management.

Cultural and Spiritual Considerations
Specific cultural, religious, or spiritual practices that may interfere with care should be shared with your social worker or medical provider (for example, a Jehovah's Witness who does not wish to receive blood transfusions).

Advanced Directives
Living wills and durable powers of attorney should be considered but are not required. An unmarried adult with no adult children should especially consider appointing a surrogate decision maker.

Institutional Support
The University of Michigan LVAD Program has two full time clinical social workers who possess Masters Degrees in social work and have combined experience exceeding 25 years. Their role consists of initial psychosocial assessment of the patient and the primary caregiver. They also provide ongoing assessment and support of the patient and family through these resources:
- *Outpatient Clinic visits*
- *Inpatient visits*

- *Peer Visitors:* patients who have undergone LVAD implant, and(or) their caregivers, and have completed specialized training by the social work staff to enable them to meet with new patients in order to orient and support them through their LVAD experience
- *Psychiatric referrals* for identified needs
- *Monthly Support Group* for Pre and Post LVAD and Transplant Patients and their Families with speakers on specific treatment related topics
- *Quarterly Newsletter* aimed at keeping patients and their caregiver(s) apprised of U-M LVAD patient activities
- *Winter and Summer Social Events:* the purpose of which is to connect patients with their peers as well as recognize them and their caregiver(s) for their courage
- *Limited Financial Resources:* to help meet the occasional transportation, lodging or meal needs for qualified patients

Online Resources

www.thoratec.com

www.mylvad.com

www.hearthope.com

Photo Pages

About this Book

In participation with Learning Design and Publishing, this initiative is based on the principle that public universities have a responsibility to share the knowledge and resources they create with the public they serve.

Based on literature of the storytelling process, this project has provided an avenue for patients who underwent LVAD implants to share their uniquely individual stories with others.

Twenty-five patients who underwent LVAD implants between July 1998 and February 2015 were recruited to share their stories of living with an LVAD. Written invitations to 25 patients resulted in submission of 17 manuscripts. Participants were required to sign a Transfer of Copyright Contract, giving the Medical School permission to publish their work.

Fourteen males and three females with ages ranging from 21 years to 72 years at time of implant submitted manuscripts. Ten are Caucasian, four are Asian and three are African American. One story was submitted by the family of their deceased sister. Copy was submitted in handwritten and typed formats, in both electronic and hard copy forms. Nine of the participants eventually underwent heart transplants, four are destination patients, one participant is still waiting for transplant, one was explanted and one destination patient is deceased.

The manuscripts were edited and published by Learning Design and Publishing, a unit within the University of Michigan Health Information Technology and Services department.

Heart 2 Heart is available for purchase from Amazon in both paperback and electronic formats.

Select stories will be available online from Open Michigan, a University collaborative committed to open content and supporting the use, redistribution, and adaptation of educational materials.

Once published, this collection of stories will also be shared with new pre LVAD candidates as a method of preparation for their own surgeries.

Thank you.

Department Events

At the University of Michigan Center for Circulatory Support, LVAD patients discover a warm environment where they and their families are supported through excellent health care. Here are some examples of recent events and materials the Center for Circulatory Support provided for LVAD and Transplant patients and their families.

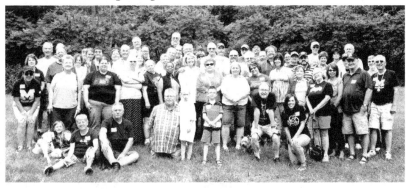

Annual Patient Picnic, a partially catered gathering where patients share their favorite dishes and experiences. One of two events at which new LVAD and Transplant patients are recognized with Olympic-type medals. Caregivers are recognized with their own lapel pin (see photo).

Family Directory

Annual Patient Directory which includes those LVAD and Transplant patients wishing to share their personal contact information with other patients. It is distributed to all patients for the benefit of communication when face-to-face contact is not possible

Caregivers Pin, created to honor the role that caregivers play in the lives of their loved ones and in our programs.

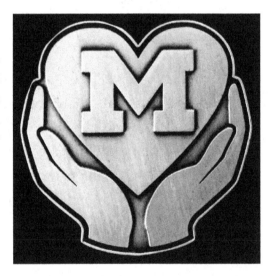

Hearts on Ice

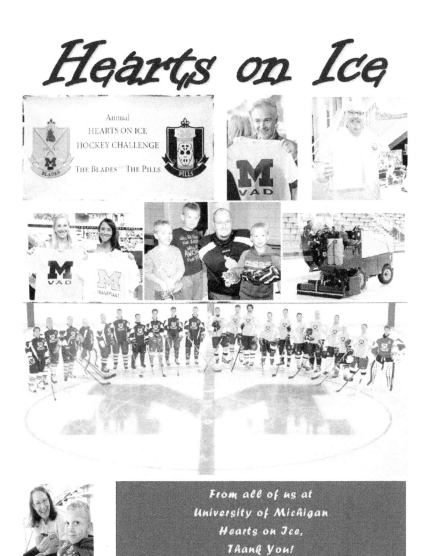

From all of us at
University of Michigan
Hearts on Ice,
Thank You!

Hearts on Ice, our annual fundraiser, supports all of
our patient programming

Annual Holiday Happening, a catered event where patients again gather to share their experiences. The second of two events at which new LVAD and Transplant recipients and their caregivers are recognized with the patient medal and caregiver lapel pin.

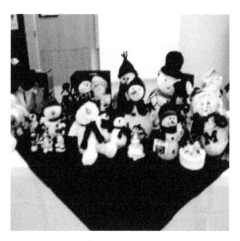

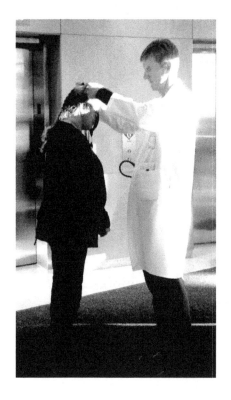

Patient Medal Presentation for LVAD and Transplant patients; Todd Koelling, M.D., one of our ten heart failure and transplant cardiologists making this presentation

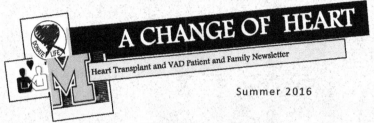

A CHANGE OF HEART

Heart Transplant and VAD Patient and Family Newsletter

Summer 2016

C a r e g i v e r s R e c o g n i z e d

For those who find themselves in the role of Caregiver, you are among 43.5 million in the United States today whose life may have changed, perhaps dramatically. It can mean a tremendous number of new responsibilities along with the emotional components of providing support and reassurance. And you share one very important thing: the service you provide, usually without benefit of professional training enables your loved one to remain at home or, in the case of transplant and LVAD consideration, actually give them the chance to live.

More inside, see 'pages 4 & 5.

Michigan Patients Waiting for a Transplant	
Heart	132
Lung	86
Liver	387
Kidney	2899
Kidney/Pancreas	60
Pancreas	23
Intestine	1
Other Organ Combos	45
TOTAL	3582

In 2015, the generosity of Michigan's 285 organ donors resulted in more than

The "Change of Heart" newsletter is yours to enjoy with your fellow heart transplant and VAD patients. It provides a place to share your special moments, suggestions, and ideas. Your stories are important to all of us, such as meeting your donor family, special events (weddings, births, anniversaries, new jobs), special talents, and important bits of information that can benefit all of us. Send your stories, ideas or comments to:

Ruth Halben, LMSW	(734) 763-9788	rhalben@umich.edu
Erin Spangler, LMSW	(734) 615-7625	espangle@umich.edu
Rebecca Congdon, LMSW	(734) 764-6205	rikera@umich.edu

If you prefer not to receive our communications, please contact Ruth, Erin or Rebecca.

Give thanks. Give life.

Patient Newsletter, published quarterly to keep both LVAD and Transplant patients informed of upcoming events and happenings of the program

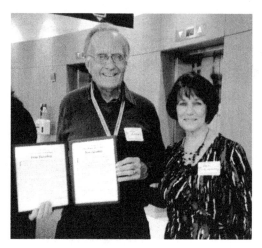

Peer Mentor of the Year, Tom Zasadny and his wife, Geri. Tom was honored by the U-M Transplant Center for 20 years of service as a Peer Visitor

Patient Medals, as mentioned, these are awarded to LVAD and Transplant patients in recognition of their courage and bravery at two annual social events

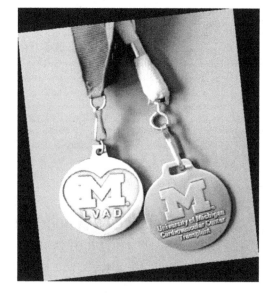

About the Editor

Ruth Halben is the fourth of eight children. She has owned a construction business, been a 911 dispatcher and managed a medical practice. In 1991 she left her job as a director of advertising for an ABC Broadcasting owned newspaper, to return to school and finish a long sought after degree. To that point, all of her education was in advertising, marketing and management from various schools of business. Upon entering the University of Michigan – Flint, 18 of her 121 credits would transfer. When asked what area of study she would pursue, her response was, 'I want to help people.' She was advised that psychology was a broad field she might want to explore.

Nearing the end of her psychology degree, she enrolled in an introductory social work class. She completed her studies with honors in 1995 and earned a B.A. with psychology and social work emphasis and a minor in Health Care Education. She interned for one year at a hospice. That fall, she began her studies at University of Michigan – Ann Arbor in the School of Social Work. While completing her Master of Social Work degree in 1996 with a Certification in Aging Studies, she also completed an internship at University of Michigan Hospital in the Heart and Lung Transplant Programs.

In January 1997, she began her professional social work career at Lapeer County Health Department Home Care Division working as a clinical social worker until December 1998. The first six months of that time were combined with a part time, temporary appointment to the Heart Transplant Program at U-M.

From May 1997 to September 1997, she collaborated with her former preceptor, Oliva Kuester, MSW on a presentation of their work on the impact of groups on patient self-care at the Society for Transplant Social workers in September 1997.

Since July 1998, Ruth has been a permanent employee of the University of Michigan Hospital in the heart transplant program and is now primarily an LVAD social worker, one of the first in this specialty area in the country. She has presented several times to the Society for Transplant Social Workers as well as given other health care related talks. Twice nominated for the Beverly Jean Howard Award for Excellence in Social Work, she has developed several social support programs, including this book, as fundamental components of her practice.

Ruth has been a field instructor for the University of Michigan School of Social Work and continues to work as a host for the School of Language, Science and Arts in the Health Science Scholars Program.

She has also worked as a home care and hospice social worker as well as provided consulting services on the social work role in home care and hospice. She has served on many boards and volunteers with the American Red Cross.

Ruth is the proud mother of three married children, grandmother to eight and great grandmother to four with another on the way. The Panda is her favorite endangered species, representative of her daughter Andrea who died of Cystic Fibrosis at the age of 15 in 1987. Ruth is an avid Michigan fan and works as an Event Staff Usher for Michigan Football and Basketball.

Go Blue!

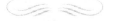

37333420R00076

Made in the USA
Middletown, DE
25 February 2019